Patients of the State

Patients of the State

THE POLITICS OF WAITING IN ARGENTINA

Javier Auyero

DUKE UNIVERSITY PRESS
Durham & London 2012

© 2012 Duke University Press
All rights reserved
Printed in the United States of America
on acid-free paper ∞
Designed by Jennifer Hill
Typeset in Garamond Premier Pro by
Keystone Typesetting, Inc.

Library of Congress
Cataloging-in-Publication Data
appear on the last printed page of
this book.

Royalties for this book are being
donated to Partners in Health.

Para Gabriela, por todo

With the coming of the Second World War, many eyes in imprisoned Europe turned hopefully, or desperately, toward the freedom of the Americas. Lisbon became the great embarkation point. But not everybody could get to Lisbon directly, and so, a tortuous, roundabout refugee trail sprang up. Paris to Marseilles, across the Mediterranean to Oran, then by train, or auto, or foot, across the rim of Africa to Casablanca in French Morocco. Here, the fortunate ones, through money, or influence, or luck, might obtain exit visas and scurry to Lisbon, and from Lisbon to the New World. But the others wait in Casablanca—and wait—and wait—and wait.

Casablanca, screenplay by Julius J. Epstein, Philip G. Epstein, and Howard Koch

For years now I have heard the word "Wait!" It rings in the ear of every Negro with piercing familiarity. This "Wait" has almost always meant "Never." We must come to see . . . that "justice too long delayed is justice denied."

MARTIN LUTHER KING JR., "Letter from Birmingham Jail"

CONTENTS

ACKNOWLEDGMENTS

Unbeknownst to my colleague Débora Swistun, this book was first conceived in a conversation with her. Thank you, Débora, for planting the seed. Once I began thinking about waiting, I needed a site to conduct the research, and my dear friend Esteban suggested a few. Esteban, it's all your fault. Agustín Burbano de Lara, Nadia Finck, and Shila Vilker were not only diligent research assistants but, most importantly, intellectual partners. This book draws upon many of the conversations I had with them over the years. I would also like to extend my heartfelt thanks to my current research collaborator, Flavia Bellomi. She not only provided key material for this book but also constantly forces me to think harder and clearer about the plight of the urban poor and about the larger implications of what we do as social scientists.

Megan Comfort, Matthew Desmond, Lauren Joseph, Rodrigo Hobert, Nicolette Manglos, Loïc Wacquant, and Christine Williams commented on parts of this manuscript. Thanks to all of you for your critical insights. Luciana Pol at Centro de Estudios Legales y Sociales kindly shared statistics on prison population and her numerous insights on the dynamics behind the explosive growth of incarceration; Christian Gruenberg helped me in locating hard-to-find figures on evictions; Nicolette Manglos, Nicole Angotti, and Pamela Neumann edited parts of this manuscript and made very helpful (substantive and stylistic) suggestions—deep thanks to you all. Generous funding for this project was provided by the National Science Foundation, Award SES-0739217; by two Andrew W. Mellon Foundation Faculty Travel Grants awarded by the Teresa Lozano Long Institute of Latin American Studies (LLILAS) and by the Joe R. and Teresa Lozano Long Professorship. Since I moved to Austin, Paloma Diaz, LLILAS's senior program coordinator, has been a wonderful *compañera*; as a steady source of ideas and an instant problemsolver, she made me work harder and better—all the while being an endless source of fun. Thanks to her for making my (and my family's) life in Austin and at the University of Texas such a wonderful experience. Thanks also to the former and current chairs of the Department of Sociology, Robert Hummer and Christine Williams, for making sure that my transition to my new academic home was as smooth as possible and for allowing me the time to work on this book amid a very demanding academic environment.

I presented parts of this book at the conference Violence in Latin America: New Realities, Emerging Representations, which was organized by the Lozano Long Institute of Latin American Studies at the University of Texas, Austin. I also presented parts at the Global Metropolitan Studies Lecture Series at the University of California, Berkeley; at the Anthropology Department of the University of Pennsylvania; at the Simon Fraser University's Latin American Studies Center; at the Facultad de Comunicación Social at the Universidad de La Plata; at the Seminario Permanente de Investigación Cualitativa (Instituto de Investigaciones Gino Germani, Universidad de Buenos Aires); and at the 2010 annual meeting of the American Sociological Association. Thanks to audiences at these diverse forums for their encouragement and comments.

Very early drafts of chapters 2 and 3 were published in *Latin American Research Review*, *Sociological Forum*, and the *European Review of Latin American and Caribbean Studies/Revista Europea de Estudios Latinoamericanos y del Caribe*; thanks to the editors and reviewers for their helpful feedback and for their permission to reproduce parts of them. I would also like to acknowledge Warner Bros. Entertainment Inc. for its permission to reproduce the quote from the opening scene of *Casablanca*, and Beacon Press for their permission to reproduce excerpts from Dr. Martin Luther King Jr.'s "Letter from Birmingham Jail" (Writings of Martin Luther King, Jr. Copyright © 2010 by the Estate of Martin Luther King, Jr. Reprinted by permission of Beacon Press, Boston).

INTRODUCTION | Tempography

🙞Waiting Now and Then

"I've been after my pension for five years now ... people at the municipal office said they lost my documents. They made me wait for a long time; they refused to see me. They gave me the run around." Silvia spent half an hour describing to me in detail all her *trámite* (paperwork), going over the different administrative levels—from municipal to federal— involved in the strenuous achievement of her meager pension: "This guy told me one thing, and then disappeared ... and then I went to the municipal office and they told me to come back in six months. And then this politician in the neighborhood told me he would take care of it but then he didn't do anything and . . ." This was 1995; Silvia was living in an extremely deprived section of a shantytown in the outskirts of Buenos Aires, and I was conducting ethnographic fieldwork for my doctoral dissertation, which later became the book *Poor People's Politics*. At the time, I was not primarily interested in Silvia's grueling pilgrimage through state bureaucracies, but rather in what and who speeded up the process. As Silvia noted further: "I began to participate in Andrea's Unidad Básica [grassroots office of the Peronist Party] and she gave me a hand. If nobody pushes these things [referring to her pension], you don't get them. Andrea was really good. If I have a problem now, I go to see her ... We have to be thankful to her; if she asks me to attend a [party] rally, I go."

Silvia's testimony was one of dozens that I used for my analysis of the workings of Peronist problem-solving "clientelist" networks. These testimonies told of the services and favors traded between clients like Silvia and brokers like Andrea, of the ways in which these exchanges are experienced, and of the long-lasting relations that ensue.

At the time, I listened and analyzed Silvia's story of her long, meandering journey through state offices *not* as a narrative that was sociologically appealing in and of itself but as a setup for what was back then my main empirical concern: brokers and their actions, and clients and their ways of reciprocating. Because of my interest in political domination, the relational object I constructed was centered on the material and symbolic exchanges between patrons, brokers, and clients. It was not, however, focused on the waiting that Silvia and many others were constantly forced to undergo in order to obtain what was rightfully theirs. These acts of waiting five years for a paltry pension and being forced to endure the runaround by state officials and local politicians did not catch my attention, even though I now understand them as *temporal processes in and through which political subordination is reproduced.* More "real" (i.e., observable, measurable) elements such as material resources, personal favors, votes, and attendance at rallies constituted my empirical universe. With the benefit of hindsight, I now see this as a missed opportunity to improve my analysis of the cultural dynamics of political clientelism. Time, its veiling and its manipulation, was and still is a key symbolic dimension in the workings of this seemingly perennial political arrangement. By ignoring this, I missed the chance for a superior understanding of political patronage.

A few years later, and in part motivated by criticisms that *Poor People's Politics* lacked attention to collective action, I embarked on a comparative qualitative study of two episodes of massive contentious politics, which formed the basis for my book *Contentious Lives.* Very much impressed by the cycle of transgressive protest in my home country of Argentina, and caught in the somewhat misleading dichotomy between clientelist and contentious politics that still pervades much of the literature (Auyero, Lapegna, and Page 2009), I initially deemed these episodes to be the opposite of the kind of patronage politics unveiled in my first book. Laura, the leader of an emblematic contentious episode and one of the main characters of the book, took many hours to re-create the aftermath of the *pueblada*, a highly disruptive protest undertaken by the residents of the towns of Cutral-co and Plaza Huincul in 1996. One night, in the home of a friend of Laura where I was staying while in Cutral-co, Laura's daughter Paula told me the following: "Right after *la pueblada*, my own house was a mess, people came at any time asking if Laura could get this and that for them." In the weeks immediately following the protest, picketers, as the protesters came to be known, attempted to organize themselves; but this time it was not to blockade roads during days and nights but to distribute the subsidies and food rations that the national and provincial governments were slowly beginning to send to town. The federal government asked the picketers' organizations to distribute state resources to the aggrieved residents. When I lived at Laura's house between January and March 2001, she described to me in detail all the *idas y venidas* (comings and goings) and all the trámites involved in delivering the promises that authorities had made to put an end to the protest. She told of meetings, long waits, more meetings, more long waits, and finally the meeting of some of their demands through work programs, subsidies, food rations, and the like.

While doing research for and writing *Contentious Lives*, I was interested in documenting the processes and mechanisms at the root of this particular form of contention, and in chronicling the ways in which Laura came to participate and make sense of this particular episode. In the book I drew upon and extended the work of C. Wright Mills to call this dynamic the intersection of biography and contention. The long delays that protesters endured after making themselves heard loud and clear on the cold roads of the Patagonian desert, and the time between the end of the protest and the partial satisfaction of the protesters' demands (or the "outcomes" to use the language of social movement scholarship), once again did not call for my sociological attention.

It took more years of fieldwork and writing for me to begin to make the empirical and theoretical connections between Silvia's and Laura's stories of waiting. These connections slowly began to emerge while doing fieldwork for the book *Flammable* (2009), which I cowrote with the anthropologist Débora Swistun. In one of the last chapters of that book we used the mythical image of Tiresias to describe one of the

defining features of the lives of the residents living in the highly contaminated shantytown called Flammable.[1] Like the Greek seer, they
are forced to become "mere onlookers of happenings beyond their
control" (Schutz 1964: 280). Shanty residents *are always waiting for
something to happen.* Those poisoned outcasts, we argue in the book,
are living in a time oriented to and manipulated by powerful agents.
They live in an alienated time, and are obliged, as Pierre Bourdieu so
eloquently puts it, "to wait for everything to come from others" (2000:
237). Domination works, we contend, through yielding to the power
of others; and it is experienced as a waiting time: waiting hopefully and
then frustratedly for others to make decisions, and in effect surrendering to the authority of others. In unexpected ways we found many versions of the Tiresias story among contemporary shantytown dwellers.

While putting the finishing touches to the manuscript I came to
realize that even if the particular and somewhat extreme relationship
between time, behavior, and submission dissected there is peculiar to
Flammable, this dynamic may be more generally applicable to all powerless groups. I then began to skim through my old fieldnotes and
progressively realized that I had not been attending to relevant parts of
what my main characters wanted me to hear: when dealing with state
authorities they were at crucial times compelled to endure lengthy
waits, were given the runaround, or were, as many subjects termed it,
"kicked around."

In shuttling back and forth between old and recent fieldnotes, I was
somewhat surprised by the number of unanalyzed moments and stories of waiting that I either experienced along with actors or which
they recollected during interviews. I began to sketch out a "tempography of domination": a thick description of how the dominated perceive temporality and waiting, how they act or fail to act on these
perceptions, and how these perceptions and these (in)actions serve to
challenge or perpetuate their domination.[2] To make the project more
manageable, I opted to concentrate on places where the urban poor
await services from the state, such as lines and waiting rooms. I also
decided to revisit my collaborative ethnography in Flammable, adding
new evidence in what resulted in a combination of revisit and re-

analysis (Burawoy 2009). My ultimate goal became to study the ways in which waiting, behavior, and submission are connected.

The results of this two-year tempography are presented in this book, *Patients of the State*. In more than one way, this book is the continuation of a research agenda that I began a decade and a half ago with *Poor People's Politics*. This agenda's main theoretical and empirical concern has been the workings of political domination among the urban poor, with a focus on its objective underpinnings and its subjective effects.

Economic globalization and neoliberal hegemony notwithstanding, the downsized, decentralized, and "hollowed out" state (Steinmetz 1999; Jessop 1999; Robinson 2008) is still a key actor in the lives of the destitute. As I illustrate below, even when the Argentine state is badly functioning and lacking in basic resources, it still has particular capacities. It grants access to citizenship, provides limited but vital welfare benefits, and exerts violence to control unruly behavior. Among the poor it is, as Akhil Gupta notes, deeply "implicated in the minute texture of everyday life" (1995: 375). Retrenched and fragmented, the state also provides powerful cultural representations. In other words, to adapt from Gilbert Joseph and Daniel Nugent's now-classic text on state-making processes in Latin America (1994), the Argentine state provides the *idiom* according to which subordinated groups initiate or fail to initiate their collective struggles. The empirical focus of this book is the relational practices linking daily state operation with the lives of the subordinate. Because, as Gupta notes, they give "concrete shape and form to what would otherwise be an abstraction ('the state')" (1995: 378), everyday encounters with state bureaucracies are central to the routine construction of the state (see also Gupta 2005; Secor 2007).

These relational practices are *cultural processes* (Steinmetz 1999; Joseph and Nugent 1994). States "state" with words, signs, and resources (Sayer 1994; Roseberry 1994), and they do so through "concrete social relations and the establishment of routines, rituals, and institutions that 'work in us'" (Joseph and Nugent 1994: 20). Thus, rather than being just a more or less functional bureaucratic apparatus, the state is also a powerful site of cultural and symbolic production (Yang 2005). States, in other words, "define and create certain kinds of subjects and identities" (Roseberry 1994: 357). They do this not simply through their police forces and armies—or what I call the "visible fists"—but also through "[their] offices and routines, [their] taxing, licensing, and registering procedures and papers" (Roseberry 1994: 357). This book thus joins in the call toward a relational analysis of political processes (Tilly 1997a; Heller and Evans 2010) that focuses on the state's day-to-day engagement with the urban poor.

For more than a decade, the social sciences have recognized the ways in which the daily practices of ordinary people construct the state (Yang 2005; Gupta 1995, 2005). Numerous studies examine the state "from the standpoint of everyday practices and the circulation of representations" (Gupta 2005: 28; see also Joseph and Nugent 1994; Gupta 1995; Yang 2005). These studies tell us that institutional forms, organizational structures, and capacities are indeed important, but so is what the state *means* to the people who inhabit it. And these meanings are constituted out of "files, orders, memos, statistics, reports, petitions, inspections, inaugurations, and transfers, the humdrum routines of bureaucracies and bureaucrats' encounters with citizens," which remain "remarkably under-studied in contrast to the predominant focus on the machinations of state leaders, shifts in major policies, regime changes, or the class basis of state officials" (Gupta 2005: 28).

The state is thereby both an abstract, macro-level structure and a concrete, micro-level set of institutions with which the urban poor interact in direct and immediate ways. In the pages that follow I will concentrate on this second level, on the level of *state practice*, by focusing on poor people's routine encounters with the state. This grounded, interactive approach to the state (Haney 1996) will allow us to examine the ways in which the state patterns both class and gender relations.

To perform this work I will personify the state and its different institutions in what Lipsky famously called "street-level bureaucrats": that is, public employees who "interact directly with individual citizens in the course of their jobs" (1980: 3). Joe Soss, in writing about encounters between these bureaucrats and applicants for AFDC (Aid to Families with Dependent Children) in the United States, points out that in these interactions bureaucrats "try to teach newcomers the expectations and obligations that will make up the 'client role'" (1999: 51). His argument underscores the relevance of clients' viewpoints in the process. It can be applied to all sorts of interactions between the destitute and the state and certainly resonates with the findings of this study. He asserts:

> Client evaluations of application encounters are politically significant... These evaluations can dissuade citizens from claiming welfare benefits—a critical form of political action for many disadvantaged groups. Eligible people may be deterred if they come to believe that the application process is too arduous and degrading or that their claims are unwanted and unlikely to succeed. If they begin to suspect that welfare clients are routinely abused and humiliated, would-be applicants may conclude that no amount of assistance is adequate compensation for joining their ranks. (51)

The recognition that through interactions between the poor and the street-level bureaucrats the state "*teaches political lessons* contributing to future political expectations" (Lipsky 1984; my emphasis) as well as socializes "citizens to expectations of government services and a place in the political community" (Lipsky 1980: 4) is central to the argument I make in this book. In their apparent ordinariness, state practices provide the poor with political education or daily crash courses on the workings of power. In the language of public administration scholars: "The conditions of application encounters can deter or facilitate demands on government. They also serve to shape clients' perceptions of their own status and authority in relation to state institutions and personnel. Consequently, clients' assessments of their application encounters provide an important subjective indicator of governmental responsiveness, measuring the quality of social citizenship" (Soss 1999: 83; see also Lens 2007). For the poor in particular, as Anna Secor notes, "the state in everyday life provokes running around uselessly and waiting," and this "ritual can best be short-circuited through the pulls" of influential personal networks (2007: 41). To recognize this is to make "a mundane observation," to paraphrase Secor's analysis of everyday practices of state power in Turkey. And yet, she states, "these quotidian stories of waiting all day only to be told to go to another office, of 'go today, come tomorrow,' of only if you know someone will you get results, provide a critical insight into *the everyday sociospatial constitution of power—not despite but because of their banality*" (42; my emphasis). Waiting lines therefore offer an excellent opportunity to study the daily exercise or denial of rights, as the anthropologist James Holston states in his study of "insurgent citizenship" in São Paulo's urban periphery. In his words:

> Standing in line for services is a privileged site for studying performances of citizenship, because it entails encounters between anonymous others in public space that require the negotiation of powers, rights, and vulnerabilities. Surely, such encounters are mundane. But trafficking in public space is a realm of modern society in which city residents most frequently and predictably experience the state of their citizenship. The quality of such mundane interaction may in fact be more significant to people's sense of themselves in society than the occasional heroic experiences of citizenship like soldiering and demonstrating of the emblematic ones like voting and jury duty. (2008: 15)

In such routine and mundane interactions citizens can demand "respect and equality," assert their "rights in public and to the public," and realign "class, gender, and race in the calculations of public standing" (17); or, in contrast, they can remain "submissive" and "powerless" (16). Properly inspected, these interactions are actually far from mundane, and they can be constructed as an extraordinary sociological object that places subjects' experiences of rights and power at the center of inquiry. Such is precisely my goal in this book. My main argument is that far from being a negative practice that merely tells poor people it is not yet their turn, making the dispossessed wait has some "possible positive effects, even if these seem marginal at first sight"

(Foucault 1979: 23). Chief among these positive effects is the everyday manufacturing of subjects who know, and act accordingly, that when dealing with state bureaucracies they have to *patiently comply with* the seemingly arbitrary, ambiguous, and always changing state requirements. Indeed, the Latin root of the word patience, which means "the quality of being patient in suffering" according to the *Oxford English Dictionary*, is *pati*: "to suffer, to endure." In the recursive interactions with the state that I chronicle in the following pages, poor people learn that they have to remain temporarily neglected, unattended to, or postponed. The poor comply because they do not have an alternative; but, as we will see by looking closely at diverse scenes of waiting, they comply silently, if begrudgingly, because they also learn that there is no use in protesting publicly. My comparative ethnographic work in three different "waiting sites" portrays poor people who *know* through repeated encounters that if they are to obtain the much needed "aid" (i.e., a welfare benefit, a service, or some other good), they have to show that they are worthy of it by dutifully waiting. They *know* that they have to avoid making trouble, and they *know*, as many people told me, that they have to "keep coming and wait, wait, wait."

The urban poor, in their frequent encounters with politicians, bureaucrats, and officials, *learn to be patients of the state*. In recurrently being forced to accommodate and yield to the state's dictates, the urban poor thereby receive a subtle, and usually not explicit, daily lesson in political subordination. Interpreted in this light, waiting ceases to be "dead time"; and making the poor wait turns into something more than a mere "repressive" action. The subjective experience of waiting and the regular practice of making the destitute wait become *productive phenomena* in need of further scrutiny. In the vein of Michel Foucault's and Pierre Bourdieu's writings, I will argue by way of demonstration that the implicit knowledge incarnated in these patients of the state reveals acts of cognition that are, simultaneously, acts of recognition of the established political order. The larger analytical lesson is therefore that habitual exposure to long delays molds a particular submissive set of dispositions among the urban poor.

"This," says Paula, "has been the longest wait." She is referring to her application to a welfare program known as Nuestras Familias. "I've been in this since March (it's now September). They asked me to come many times; there was always something (a document, a paper) missing." Paula tells her daughter Nana that, if she behaves well, she will take her to the nearby park as "her prize" for spending so many hours in the waiting room. "It is really exhausting [fatigoso] to wait here; I'm lucky because she (Nana) behaves really well." When Paula comes to the welfare office, she tells us, "you have to be calm, to be patient." Although she has seen other beneficiaries expressing their anger against welfare agents, "I never ever get mad, I'm always calm. Here, you have to have patience. This is an aid that the government gives you, so you have to be patient."

For reasons that will become clear as my analysis progresses, it is not easy to investigate the waiting of the dispossessed. I anchor my study in three main physical spaces: the Registro Nacional de las Personas (RENAPER), where legal residents of Argentina apply for a national ID card; the welfare agency of the city of Buenos Aires; and the shantytown of Flammable where, together with a team of research collaborators, I conducted extensive ethnographic fieldwork. In the methodological appendix to this book I describe these diverse fieldwork experiences as well as the guide used to observe and then interview people waiting in line in both the welfare agency and the RENAPER. As in previous work (Auyero and Swistun 2009), my collaborators and I follow the evidentiary criteria normally used for ethnographic research (Becker 1958; Katz 1982), which assigns higher evidentiary value to the conduct we were able to observe versus the behavior reported by interviewees to have occurred and to the patterns of conduct recounted by many observers versus those recounted by a single one.

Most of the interactions analyzed in the pages that follow were witnessed firsthand by me or by my collaborators. In that sense, this work can be defined as ethnographic in the classic sense of the term (Geertz 1973; Burawoy et al. 1991). A very basic, agreed-upon definition of ethnography, spelled out by Loïc Wacquant, is as follows: "[It is] social research based on the close-up, on-the-ground observation of people and institutions in real time and space, in which the investigator embeds herself near (or within) the phenomenon so as to detect how and why agents on the scene act, think and feel the way they do" (2003b: 5).

Poor people "experience deprivation and oppression within a concrete setting, not as the end product of large and abstract processes" (Piven and Cloward 1978: 20). Their concrete experiences in specific social universes are the objects of our ethnographic inquiry in this study. They matter because the destitute in our work do not experience "neoliberalism" or "globalization" in a strict sense, but rather shabby waiting rooms, uncomfortable lines, endless delays, and meager and random welfare benefits (Piven and Cloward 1978). We joined our subjects in these rooms and lines, as well as in some of their homes, in an attempt to reconstruct their views and experiences of waiting.

We witnessed interactions between poor dwellers and state agents unfolding and were effectively "immersed in" (Schatz 2009) the processes under investigation, whether they be the acquisition of an ID card, the granting of a welfare subsidy, or the expected relocation of a neighborhood. As witnesses, we did our best to understand and explain the actions, thoughts, and feelings of the parties involved.

In all the interactions under scrutiny, at least one of the parties was a government agent; so in this sense, our ethnography was political (Auyero and Joseph 2008; Schatz 2009). Charles Tilly (cited in Auyero 2008) once described political ethnography as a

> risky business, at once intensely sociable and deeply isolating. On one side, its effective pursuit requires close involvement with political actors, and therefore the danger of becoming their dupes, their representatives, their brokers, or their accomplices. On the other, bringing out the news so others can understand depends on multiple translations: from the stories that political participants tell into stories that audiences will understand, from local circumstances to issues that will be recognizable outside the locality, from concrete

explanations for particular actions to accounts in which outsiders will at least recognize analogies to classes of actions with which they are familiar.

Tilly's forthright assertion became a stimulating invitation as I embarked in this project. As much as any of the other research in which I have been involved in the past two decades, this project challenged me to find a balance between involvement and detachment, between the personal and the systematic, between being there among the waiting populace and being here among academics, between stories told in the field and stories told to the public, and between describing personal dramas and achieving sound sociological explanations.

Over the years, I have been undertaking a kind of political ethnography that intended to critically evaluate the strengths and limitations of central sociological concepts such as clientelism, power, legitimacy, habitus, mobilizing structures, and so forth (Auyero 2000, 2003, 2007). By demonstrating the adequacy (or inadequacy) of these conceptual tools vis-à-vis a detailed description of the processes they are meant to describe, my work has attempted to show the virtues and shortcomings of these key concepts. This testing of the adequacy of concepts against the empirical reality identifies the risks involved in an uncritical application of such concepts, and clears the way for the development of more precise concepts and theories that provide a better fit with empirical data. While this sort of political ethnography seldom is able to directly test theoretical hypotheses, it is essential to a critical appraisal of the capability of the central organizing concepts employed by those who wish to test theories against empirical data.[3] All too often, I should add, such theory testing is performed on what might be termed "stylized facts"—oversimplified descriptions generated by concepts and notions that usually fail to capture the fine-grained microsociological processes at work. As a result, much macrosociological work in political sociology rests on conceptually weak microfoundations. All in all, the kind of political ethnography I undertake (and advocate for) is an essential tool to provide a more solid foundation for sociological work (both theoretical and empirical).

Ethnography is uniquely equipped to look microscopically at the foundations of political institutions and their attendant practices, just as it is ideally suited to dissect politics' day-to-day intricacies (Baiocchi 2005) and implicit meanings (Lichterman 1998). The ethnographic reconstructions presented here might seem personal, anecdotal, banal, or idiosyncratically focused on a malfunctioning state in the periphery of the world system. Yet the relational object constructed out of the trivial, ordinary, and context specific is, I hope, one that should be of interest to those who examine the domination of subaltern populations in other times and settings.

"With one quick look," writes Jorge Luis Borges in "Funes, His Memory,"

> you and I perceive three wineglasses on a table; Funes perceived every grape that had been pressed into the wine and all the stalks and tendrils of its vineyard. He knew the forms of the clouds in the southern sky on the morning of April 30, 1882, and he could compare them in his memory with the veins in the marbled binding of a book he had seen only once, or with the feathers of spray lifted by an oar on the Río Negro on the eve of the Battle of Quebracho. (1999: 135)

Ireneo Funes had a prodigious memory. He "remembered not only every leaf of every tree in every patch of forest, but every time he had perceived or imagined that leaf" (135), but he was utterly incapable of general ideas. "Not only was it difficult for him to see that the generic symbol 'dog' took in all the dissimilar individuals of all shapes and sizes, it irritated him that the 'dog' of three-fourteen in the afternoon, seen in profile, should be indicated by the same noun as the dog of three-fifteen, seen frontally" (136). Despite his meticulous memory, Funes was "not very good at thinking." Borges reminds us that thinking "is to ignore (or forget) differences, to generalize, to abstract. In the teeming world of Ireneo Funes there was nothing but particulars—and they were virtually all *immediate* particulars" (137).

Ethnographers venturing into the sites portrayed in this book face a dilemma similar to Funes. There are too many particulars; too many immediate concerns, stories, voices, sounds, and smells bombard us throughout our field research and obfuscate our vision. To make matters worse, many of these are on first sight quite ordinary. How are we to see? To avoid Ireneo Funes's fate, the ethnographer needs categories or classificatory schemes to bring some order and understanding to, and then explain, the highly consequential nature of the "minor" happenings right in front of her eyes. If she is to see, the ethnographer needs at least some provisional theory. Without a theory to be revised, improved, and reconstructed, "we are blind, we cannot see the world" (Burawoy 2009). Theory helps the ethnographer to organize and to abstract from the "multiform, momentaneous, and almost unbearably precise world" of Funes. Out of the all-too-ordinary encounters and stories witnessed in diverse settings, my concern with the relationship between domination and the manipulation of time led me to focus on the relational experience of waiting. As my narrative moves forward the reader should be able to see how my provisionary theoretical point of view generates, as Gaston Bachelard would say, the empirical object to be understood and explained (2006 [1938]).

This book is not, however, based exclusively on ethnography. Other data sources were also examined in my search for "waiting experiences": court cases describing the political maneuvering behind an incident of arson in a shantytown, chronicles written by investigative journalists depicting violent evictions, human rights reports delving into cases of police violence, and newspaper stories describing poor people's interactions with different areas of the state.

In various "strategic research sites" (Merton 1987) I witnessed an almost uncontested compliance with the fundamental presuppositions of the workings of the state, or "the silence of the (waiting) doxa" (Bourdieu 1991: 51). The state tells its subjects, either implicitly or explicitly, with words or with actions: "Wait, be patient, and you might benefit from my (reluctant) benevolence." Subjects heed this injunction to wait because it is rooted in their reality. After all, they are always waiting. In our diverse research settings, waiting appears to be "in the order of things" for the poor. It is something normal, expected, and inevitable. They are disposed to recognize that they have to wait and thus to submit to it, because that is precisely what they are regularly exposed to. Waiting is neither a trait of their character nor something they "value" because they have a different appreciation of time, as a "culture of poverty" type of argument would have it; rather, it is a product of a successful strategy of domination.

ROADMAP

In the first chapter of this book I draw upon classic works of fiction, including Gabriel García Márquez's *No One Writes to the Colonel*, Samuel Beckett's *Waiting for Godot*, and Franz Kafka's *The Trial*, as well as on literature in the social sciences in order to both justify my focus on waiting and to formulate my guiding questions.

Chapter 2 is based in contemporary Argentina, and it begins with a statistical description of the nation's trends in poverty and inequality along with ethnographic vignettes depicting the daily lives of the urban poor. I then move on to examining three different forms of regulating mass misery: "visible fists" (repression, imprisonment, territorial sieges, and the like); "clandestine kicks" (illegal exercises of violence carried out by actors connected with established powerholders); and "invisible tentacles" (less obvious or violent forms of power that achieve the subordination of poor people by making them "sit and wait").

Frances Fox Piven and Richard Cloward, writing in 1971 about the uses of relief giving in regulating poor people's economic and social behavior, indicated that "relief arrangements are initiated or expanded during the occasional outbreaks of civil disorder produced by mass unemployment and are then abolished or contracted when political stability is restored" (1971: xv). The argument of their now-classic book *Regulating the Poor: The Functions of Public Welfare* is straightforward: "Expansive relief policies are designed to mute civil disorder, and restrictive ones to reinforce work norms" (xv). The mass disorders produced by labor market dislocations are dealt with relief programs that are later "retained (in an altered form) to enforce work" (xvii). In the United States these programs—provisions known as "public assistance or public welfare" (3)—are, according to the authors, the main way in which the state manages the poor:

> When mass unemployment leads to outbreaks of turmoil, relief programs are ordinarily initiated or expanded to absorb and control enough of the unemployed to restore order; then, as turbulence subsides, the relief system contracts, expelling those who are needed to populate the labor market. Relief also performs a labor-regulating function in this shrunken state, however. Some of the aged, the disabled, the insane, and others who are of no use as workers are left on the relief rolls, and their treatment is so degrading and punitive as to instill in the laboring masses a fear of the fate that awaits them should they relax into beggary and pauperism. (3)

Almost forty years after the publication of *Regulating the Poor*, Loïc Wacquant's *Punishing the Poor* (2009) signals an epochal change in the management of the destitute. As he writes, the "cyclical dynamic of expansion and contraction of public aid . . . has been superseded by a *new division of labor of nomination and domination of deviant and dependent populations* that couples welfare services and criminal justice administration under the aegis of the same behaviorist and punitive philosophy" (14, emphasis in original). Welfare disciplinary programs and an extended police and penal net are now "two components of a single apparatus for the management of poverty . . . In the era of fragmented and discontinuous wage work, the regulation of working-class households is no longer handled solely by the maternal and nurturing social arm of the *welfare state*; it relies also on the virile and controlling arm of the *penal state*" (14, emphasis added). According to Wacquant, this means that in the United States poverty regulation now takes place in public aid offices and job placement bureaus, as well as in police stations, criminal courts, and prison cells.

What Wacquant describes as a new development in the United States has been a durable feature of the modern state in Argentina and in many other Latin American countries at least since the mid-1940s. The management of mass poverty has always been carried on jointly by

the "social" arm and the "punitive" arm of the state. In various historical periods one strategy of domination has prevailed over the other,
but both have coexisted in ways analogous to Wacquant's description.
In adapting his analysis we could say that during the populist period
the dominant form of regulation tended to occur in union offices and
by those in charge of mass assistance programs, from the initiatives of
the Fundación Evita to the current jobless programs (Giraudy 2007;
Bianchi and Sanchis 1988; Navarro and Fraser 1985). During authori-
tarian times, the labor of domination took place more so in police
stations, prison cells, street repression, and in concentration camps,
especially during the last dictatorship (1976–1983) (Actis et al. 2006;
Partnoy 1998; Arditti 1999). Since the mid-1990s, as wage work started
to vanish, informal labor spread, and poverty mounted, the Argentine state has simultaneously stepped up both forms of "regulating the
poor." In chapter 2 I describe these forms in detail, and I tell the story
of one individual—a composite created out of many stories heard in
the field—to illustrate the forms of power that poor people experience
in their daily encounters with the state. The chapter ends with a rough
sketch of the workings of the less visible forms of power.

In chapter 3 I begin with an analytical reconstruction of an incident
of arson, which I use to portray both the precarious character of the
lives of shantytown dwellers in contemporary Buenos Aires and to
foreground the central place of waiting in the lives of the most vulnerable. I then turn to the story of one exemplary waiter, a kind of *Odys-
sey*'s Penelope who exists as an ideal-typical case of poor people's shared
experiences of waiting. In drawing upon four months of ethnographic
observations, I center this chapter on the process of acquiring a DNI
(*documento nacional de identidad*, or national ID card) at the offices of
the RENAPER, and anticipate the *uncertainty* and *arbitrariness* that
characterize the long delays routinely experienced by the destitute. I
also describe the three processes they are exposed to as they interact
with the state: veiling, confusion, and alternate delaying and rushing.
Chapter 4 expands on this when I delve into the Kafkaesque universe
of the welfare office of Buenos Aires. Based on one year of ethnographic fieldwork, I examine the welfare office as a site of intense so-

ciability amid a pervasive sense of puzzlement. The demands that the state regularly makes on its subjects ("sit down and wait") become quite clear here. On a daily basis, I argue, *patients of the state are being manufactured in the ordinary encounters between welfare agents and the poor*. This chapter examines the many twists and turns of a somewhat invisible exercise of power, which is quite effective precisely because of this invisibility (Lukes 2004).

In chapter 5 I return to Flammable, the neighborhood where together with the resident and anthropologist Débora Swistun I conducted ethnographic work on environmental suffering between 2004 and 2006 (Auyero and Swistun 2009). The chapter is based on a reanalysis of previous field data and on new material gathered in 2009 and early 2010. After a brief presentation of the case of "toxic waiting" experienced by residents of Ezpeleta—a neighborhood with unprecedented levels of cancer likely produced by a power transformer plant—I chronicle recent events in Flammable and examine the intimate connection between residents' experiences of waiting and their shared understandings of politics. I find, much like at the time of our original fieldwork, that neighbors are "still waiting" for relocation or eviction or indemnification. Whatever outcome brings the end of their waiting is, they believe, pretty much determined by politics; and politics is not understood as an activity that *they* do or as a motor of collective change, but rather as an alien, distant practice that renders them powerless.

In addition to developing a social science account of waiting among the poor, this book has two complementary and primarily descriptive aims: first, to depict in as complete ethnographic detail as possible the daily lives of those living at the bottom of the social structure who have extremely precarious attachments to the labor and the housing markets, and do so in a society still suffering from the consequences of a neoliberal transformation; and second, to chronicle the ways in which these dispossessed denizens interact with a state that presumably cares for their plight.

It is neither an empirical nor a theoretical surprise that poor people have to wait longer than others, and I doubt that an ethnographic analysis (much less so a book) with the main aim of providing further evidence of this general assessment would be warranted. In fact, several times when speaking in public about the subject of this book, I was confronted with puzzled looks. I was, most academic audiences seem to suggest, tackling the obvious (that poor people wait) and the perennial (that it has always been that way). The issue for me then became how we account for or *explain* the apparent eternal character of poor people's waiting. Pierre Bourdieu's work, as both a science of practice and a critique of domination, provided many of the thinking tools I used to analyze waiting as an exercise of power. Poor people's waiting shares many of the traits of masculine domination. It is inscribed in the mental and bodily dispositions of both dominant (i.e., men, state agencies) and dominated (women, those who wait), and because of this inscription both groups tend to naturalize or "eternalize" this relationship of domination. Those that are forced to endure long, routine delays come to see waiting as unavoidable, as a sort of habitual practice that is taken for granted (Garfinkel 1967). In reasoning by analogy (Vaughan 2004), I argue that in order to fully understand and explain why the destitute wait and why this waiting seems somewhat "normal" to them (and to many academics), we need to reconstruct the *daily labor of normalizing waiting*. To do so, we need a thorough and systematic inspection of the words and deeds of those who wait and those who make them wait, as well as the relationships that they establish in the process.

Going one step further, the analysis that follows also seeks to dissect the way in which this *waiting (re)creates subordination*. It does so, I argue, by *producing uncertainty and arbitrariness*. The uncertainty and arbitrariness engenders one particular subjective effect among those who need the state to survive: they silently comply (*ply* from the Latin *plicare*, to bend) with the authorities' usually capricious commands. To put it bluntly, everyday political domination is what happens when nothing apparently happens, when people "just wait."

What we witness in this indeterminate waiting is thus the daily reproduction of a mode of domination founded "on the creation of a generalized and permanent state of insecurity" (Bourdieu 1999: 85) that aims to, and to a great extent succeeds in, forcing the poor into submission. In making them wait, the state reinforces the uncertainty and the arbitrariness that is already present in poor people's daily lives. This is why waiting for the state, which is presumably the one actor that should be in charge of their welfare, is much more aggravating and consequential. At a time when governments across the region claim a renewed role for the state in correcting previous injustices and redistributing the nations' wealth, among other things, the different levels of the state analyzed here seem to be doing just the opposite. When interacting with a state that publicly presents itself as "concerned" about them, vulnerable residents should not be anxiously dreading the future. Why they do so becomes clear in the pages that follow.

Leticia is by herself, standing alone in the back of the waiting room of the welfare office. It's early in the morning, a placid sunny day in September. She left her three children (twelve, ten, and six years old) at home: "The oldest one is in charge of taking them to school. I have to spend the morning here, doing paperwork for the Nuestras Familias (NF) program." She woke up very early this morning, and her youngest daughter, seeing her getting ready to leave, asked to come along: "I told her that I was coming to the welfare office: 'Do you remember? We have to walk all the way there, wait for a long time, and then come back walking.' She immediately desisted. Last time she came, she was very bored; she was hungry, uncomfortable . . ." Today is the third time Leticia has come to this office in the last two weeks. "I'm used to waiting," she says, "I have to wait everywhere. But the worst thing is that they make you go here and then there ["te tienen de acá para allá"]. I do this for my children; if it were not for them, I wouldn't be here." She began the paperwork for the NF four months ago. "I came two weeks ago; they told me to come back in three days. I came back and the office was closed. I returned the next day, and they told me there were no funds in the program. Today I need to get paid." Leticia defines the welfare office as a place where "you have to wait, because that's how things are here. You have to come many times because if you don't show up, you don't get anything." Leticia believes that "we are all equals. There shouldn't be a difference but, well, if you have money everything is quicker . . . if not, you have to wait."

The diverse portraits offered in the following chapters cohere, I hope, into a single landscape. My intention is for this landscape to depict a particular ordinary encounter between poor people and the state as being characterized by the routine truncation or utter denial of "interactional citizenship": the "set of vague and diffuse but vitally felt expectations and obligations that pertain to interactional displays of respect, regard and dignity for the person" (Colomy and Brown 1996: 375). As part of their routine operations, state agencies disregard many of the strictures of interactional citizenship. The message conveyed by different state officials toward those obliged to wait is not one of respect but one of inferiority, and the uncertainty and arbitrariness of the delays signal the state's total disregard for the waiting populace. In making them wait for every single service for typically an unusually long time, state officials are effectively telling the poor that their time and therefore their worth is less valuable than the time and worth of others (Schwartz 1974). I argue that taken together these waiting experiences persuade the destitute that they need to be "patient," and therefore convey the implicit state request to be compliant clients. Such an analysis of the sociocultural dynamics of waiting helps us to understand how the destitute come to be defined and treated not as citizens but as patients of the state.

As Patrick Heller and Peter Evans have written, "Citizenship is always multi-scalar. Citizens are made not only at the national level through constitutions and elections, but also in their day-to-day engagements with the local state" (2010: 435). This engagement of the poor with the local political apparatus constitutes the empirical focus of this book. The *relationship* between destitute subjects and the state is of analytical and theoretical importance because it is a defining feature of the actual character of citizenship and of the workings of democracy, as well as the ensuing impact on inequality (Tilly 2006, 2007). Following Charles Tilly, Heller and Evans summarize the relationship between citizenship, democracy, and inequality as follows: "Democratization is best understood as an expansion in the quality of citizenship, which is about the institutionalized quality of a subject's relation to government and its authority, which in turn exists in in-

verse proportion to the degree to which a subject's relations to government are mediated by categorical inequalities" (435). As we will see,
categorical inequalities of class and gender mediate the relationship
between subjects and the state and hamper their exercise of citizenship.
Everyday de-democratization and expanding inequality can be seen in
the particular social universes under investigation.

Let me conclude here with the main substantive implication of the
analysis that follows. In paraphrasing Sharon Hays's analysis of welfare
mothers in the United States during the age of welfare reform (2003),
we could assert that if the state really wants to include welfare beneficiaries, shanty dwellers, and legal aliens as active citizens—that is, full-
fledged participants in society—it does not make much sense to make
them wait in the zones of uncertainty and arbitrariness described in
this book. If, on the other hand, what the state is actually doing is creating subordinate subjects who do not raise their voice, who "know"
because they learn in practice that they have to be patient, then the
uncertainty and arbitrariness that dominates the spatial and temporal
universes examined below can be viewed as a very effective route.

ONE | The Time of the Denizens

"Shit" is the last word in Gabriel García Márquez's short and moving novel *No One Writes to the Colonel* (1979). The colonel, awaiting the outcome of an upcoming cockfight, is replying to his wife who impatiently wants to know what they will eat. As the cock's owner, who is also its feeder and trainer, the colonel will be entitled to 20 percent of the winning bet. The colonel refuses to sell the rooster to pay for food. Instead, he asks his wife to wait forty-four more days and to place her trust in the rooster that "can't lose."

The colonel's reply, *mierda*, can be read as a foul response to an anxious and demanding wife. Yet the meaning of that answer transcends the specific moment in the narrative. The colonel feels "pure, explicit, and invincible" (62), Márquez tells us, because he is articulating his feelings after so many years of suffering, disappointments, frustrations, and fifteen years of waiting for the government pension to which he is entitled "after risking [his] neck in the civil war" (60). Every Friday, after visiting the postmaster, he realizes that "no one writes to the colonel." His expectations for the pension barely sustain him, and he and his wife continue to have difficulty in making ends meet, so he hangs his hopes on the rooster's victory.

Márquez's emotive tale can be read as a realistic and illustrative narrative of many people's experiences in Latin America. The governments that fail to deliver promised protection to their citizens but are swift in delivering terror against dissenters are represented in the story by the pension that never arrives and the loss of a son to state repression. The story also expresses the region's political instability: "Just think about it, [in the last fifteen years] there have been seven Presidents, and each President changes his Cabinet at least ten times, and each Minister changes his staff at least a hundred times" (26). Finally, the book can also be read as a highly perceptive account of the meanings and feelings at work in the experience of waiting. *No One Writes to the Colonel* chronicles endless waiting from the point of view of the colonel and his wife and masterfully describes the changing import of that waiting time from hopefulness to resignation. The central characters are not given names, which increases the reader's sense of their insignificance in the light of such bureaucratic indifference ("Those documents have passed through thousands and thousands of hands, in thousands and thousands of offices, before they reached God knows which department" [26]). Yet the lack of names also points to the fact that anybody can be the colonel. Never-ending waiting, sometimes hopeful, other times resigned, characterizes the lives of the dispossessed. It defines their identity, much like that of the colonel who becomes "a man with no other occupation than waiting for the mail every Friday" (17). The poor may stubbornly defend their dignity while they retain hope for a better future. But in their daily lives, "it is always the same story" (24); they are forced to wait for powerful others to make good on their promises. "Wait" is a command that, to paraphrase this book's opening quote by Martin Luther King Jr., rings in the ear of every poor person with piercing familiarity. Waiting, in other words, is a recurring, almost modal, experience among the destitute.

Waiting Inscribed in Space

"Early in the morning of October 10, 1970, in the midst of a cold rain," writes the urbanist Janice Perlman in her four-decade-long study of three *favelas* in Rio de Janeiro, "the military police and several large garbage trucks (note symbolism) arrived in front of Catacumba and proceeded to remove everyone and everything" (2010: 78). What was once a thriving community climbing up the hills facing the Lagoa Rodrigo Freitas is now the place of a "little-used park and million dollar condos" (63). Eviction was swiftly accomplished; not so much relocation of *favelados*. Fourteen hundred and twenty families were sent to the adjacent conjuntos [government-run apartment complexes] of Guaporé and Quitungo, 350 to Cidade de Deus, 87 to Vila Kennedy, and 350, too poor for apartments, were sent off to triage units in a remote area call Paciencia. . . . The families sent to the triage units found row upon row of attached one-room wooden houses in the middle of nowhere. There was no access to jobs, schools, clinics, or work. *It is only fitting that the name of the place where they were left to rot was Paciencia (Patience)*. . . . When I returned to Rio in 1973, for the first time after the [original] study was done [published as *The Myth of Marginality* (1976)], I went to Paciencia by bus—a trip of over three and a half hours—to see what it was like. I passed hundreds of acres of uncultivated lands and saw neither dwellings nor signs of commerce. What I found when we arrived was a variation on a debtors' prison, a dead end without exit. I will never forget speaking with a woman in her front door, who turned to me and asked, "Where does the end of the world end? . . . Where will they throw us, finally?" . . . Indeed, it did seem like *o fin do mundo*. The ranks of those sent to the triage housing from all of the removed favelas were further swelled by those sent there for defaulting on their monthly payments in the conjuntos. Hundreds of additional triage units were under construction when I was there in 1973—red brick boxes with corrugated metal roofs all lined up in the dry dirt, baking in the sun. (78–80; my emphasis)

In this book I offer a sociological sketch of the urban poor's experience of waiting, which is so widespread among them but has rarely been scrutinized in a systematic way. I take the reader into three different social universes in contemporary Argentina in order to dissect the meanings that usually long and sometimes endless waiting has for the underprivileged, and to examine the ways in which "making poor people wait" works as a strategy of domination.

Waiting, writes Pierre Bourdieu in *Pascalian Meditations*, is one of the privileged ways of experiencing the effects of power. The elements of "making people wait . . . delaying without destroying hope . . . adjourning without totally disappointing" (2000: 228) are, according to Bourdieu, integral to the workings of domination. Although certain links between power and time have been thoroughly examined in the social sciences, waiting—as both a temporal region and as an activity intricately bound up with the constitution and reproduction of submission—remains, with few exceptions, "hardly mapped and badly documented" (Schweizer 2008: 1; see also Gasparini 1995). This is understandable, given the preferred focus in the social sciences on individual and collective action, or on the *event* as that "historical fact that leaves a unique and singular trace, one that marks history by its particular and inimitable consequences" (Dumoulins quoted in Tarrow 1996: 587).

In writing about this inattention to waiting, Bourdieu asserts that we need to "catalogue, and analyze, all the behaviors associated with the exercise of power over other people's time both on the side of the powerful (adjourning, deferring, delaying, raising false hopes, or conversely, rushing, taking by surprise) and on the side of the 'patient,' as they say in the medical universe, one of the sites par excellence of anxious, powerless waiting" (2000: 228). In drawing upon extensive multisited ethnographic fieldwork, in this book I make a first step toward the construction of such a catalogue of poor people's waiting experiences.

TIME, POWER, AND THE (SCANT) SOCIOLOGY OF WAITING

The ways in which human beings in their lifeworlds think, feel about, and act on time have been the subject of much scholarly work in the social sciences. There have been more general treatments (Sorokin and Merton 1937; Hall 1959; Schutz 1964; Durkheim 1965; Giddens 1986; Munn 1992; Levine 1997; Flaherty 1999) as well as more empirically informed ones, many of them based on ethnographic work (Roth 1963; Mann 1969; Geertz 1973; Zerubavel 1979; Young 2004; Flaherty, Freiding, and Sautu 2005; Flaherty 2010). The relationship between the *workings of power* (Lukes 2004) and the *experiences of time* has been well studied. To name some examples, time has been examined as a crucial dimension in the workings of gift exchanges (Bourdieu 1977) and in the operation of patronage networks (Scott and Kerkvliet 1977). In both these cases, the objective truth of these usually unequal exchanges needs to be *misrecognized* so that the exchanges can function smoothly, and time is responsible for the veiling (Bourdieu 1998; Ortner 2006).

Historical and ethnographic works also illustrate that temporality is malleable. It can be the object of a "continual process of bargaining," such as when patients and doctors jointly structure the passage of time in a tuberculosis hospital (Roth 1963); or it can be the object of frantic "marking," such as occurs in the security wing of an English prison (Cohen and Taylor 1972). Time can also be the target of a constant onslaught, as Paul Willis (1977) illustrates in his dissection of the rejection by the students at one school of the school's arduously constructed timetable; or it can be the medium through which discipline is imposed and negotiated, as E. P. Thompson (1994) demonstrates in his classic analysis of the changes in the inward notations of time during the early stages of industrial capitalism. Collective time senses are deeply intertwined with both the workings of and resistance to social domination. Time is an important locus of both conflict and acquiescence (see also Hochschild 2001; Thompson and Bunderson 2001; Jacobs and Gerson 2005; Purser 2006).

Despite this ample literature, waiting has not received the same scholarly attention. In highlighting the ubiquity of this experience, the essayist Edna O'Brien writes: "Everyone I know is waiting." Hinting at the sense of powerlessness that comes with waiting, she continues by noting, "and almost everyone I know would like to rebut it, since it is slightly demeaning, reeks of helplessness, and shows we are not fully in command of ourselves" (1995: 177). With all due respect to O'Brien, waiting does not affect everybody in the same way, nor is it experienced in a similar fashion. Rather, waiting is stratified, and there are variations in waiting time that are socially patterned and responsive to power differentials (Schwartz 1974; 1975). In *Queuing and Waiting*, Barry Schwartz's now classic study of queues as social systems, the author writes: "Typical relationships obtain between the individuals' position within a social system and the extent to which he waits for and is waited for by other members of the system. In general, the more powerful and important a person is, the more others' access to him must be regulated" (1975: 847). To be kept waiting, he continues, "especially to be kept waiting an unusually long time, is to be the subject of an assertion that one's own time (and therefore, one's social worth) is less valuable than the time and worth of the one who imposes the wait" (856; see also Comfort 2008). Schwartz's book established the basic contours for a sociological analysis of waiting. Since then, however, the unequal distribution of waiting time and the activities that go with it have received scant empirical treatment.

The research that does exist shows that extensive waiting periods "weary people" (Piven and Cloward 1971: 160) and act as obstacles to accessing particular programs (Redko, Rapp, and Carlson 2006). If frequent contact with long queues truly molds people's subjectivities (Comfort 2008; Bourdieu 2000), how exactly does it happen that such efforts toward some specified end result in modifying the behaviors of those who wait? If delays are *not only suffered but also interpreted* (Schwartz 1975), what meanings do those who are routinely forced to wait attribute to the waiting? And, if waiting makes the waiter feel "dependent and subordinate" (Schwartz 1975: 856), how does waiting produce these subjective effects of dependency and subordination? In other words, how does objective waiting become subjective submission?

TWO CLASSICS ON WAITING

In stark contrast with the paucity of examinations by social scientists of the experience of waiting (on how and why people "put up" with it, and on what sorts of effects this tolerance has on their being in the world), literary renditions of waiting as a lived reality, as that "bitter, cosmic task" (Gilman 1987: 78), abound. Waiting has been the implicit or explicit subject of classic romance novels as well as of several contemporary narratives (Jin 2000; Arango 1995; Sorokin 2008). However, as I ventured into my field sites and began to think systematically about how the dominated make sense of their waiting time, two literary masterpieces became particularly inspiring to me: Samuel Beckett's *Waiting for Godot* and Franz Kafka's *The Trial*. These two works provided what Herbert Blumer would call "sensitizing devices," which first made me aware of how much goes on when people "just wait" although seemingly nothing happens; and, second, helped me realize that the experience of waiting has a processual and relational character.

According to Hugh Kenner, there is a good reason that there was never a play about waiting before Beckett's *Waiting for Godot*. "No dramatist before Beckett," Kenner writes, "ever thought of attempting such a thing. It seems contrary to the grain of the theater, where the normal unit is the event, and where intervals between events are cleverly filled so as to persuade us that the cables are weaving and tightening that shall produce the next event" (1987: 61). Dozens of essays have been written about *Waiting for Godot*, but I won't attempt to summarize their many interesting insights on the play's substance, message, impact, reception, and the like (see the essays in Bloom 1987). Rather, I want to highlight just one main element that will serve as a guide for the ethnographic inquiries that follow.

In *Waiting for Godot* we could find a paradigmatic example of waiting as a *lack of activity* . . . but with a twist. Richard Gilman puts it this way: Beckett's is "a play of absence, a drama whose binding element is what *does not take place*" (1987: 70; emphasis in original). In the play, Hugh Kenner states, there is "nothing to be done" (1987: 55), and the identities of the two main characters are defined by what they do: they are "men who must wait" (Gilman 1987: 72). Harold Schweizer emphasizes this latter dimension by pointing out that this focus on the identity of those who wait is the novelty of the play. He asserts that it centers on "how we are" in the waiting and on the "quality of waiting as such":

> When we say that in Godot we just wait, we mean that waiting has been emptied of all practical, philosophical, or theological resonance. . . . What Vladimir and Estragon wait for is perhaps only to get to—and to get us to—this literalism of waiting, to experience their waiting first and foremost, and perhaps ultimately, as nothing

other than the endurance of time. For this is not waiting for something that would validate, cancel, or fulfill waiting. This is the kind of waiting we fear that waiting—or living—might amount to: just waiting. (2008: 12)

But there would be no play if Vladimir and Estragon had not "devise[d]—it is the exact word—a provisional, tactical liberty, one of speech and small gestures. They are like prisoners free to amuse one another or to take advantage of the penitentiary's game room, the crucial difference being that for them the prison walls are as wide as the earth" (Gilman 1987: 72). And therein lies the beauty, and some would claim the success, of Beckett's play: *a lot goes on (between the main characters, between them and others) when nothing apparently happens.* That is, after all, why we have a play. This seemingly simple message ultimately became my starting point. What happens while people hang out and hang on an expected decision in the welfare office, in the outside of the RENAPER, or in the shantytown with apparently nothing else to do other than waiting for their "Godot," such as access to a welfare program, a much-needed ID, a lawyer that will bring good news? In contrast to my previous work on popular politics (Auyero 2003, 2007), in which I paid attention to "moments of madness" (Zolberg 1972) and other grand episodes of mass contention in which people break with their daily routines and make collective, public claims, here I analyze such unimportant happenings that never make it to the news.

It is true that the habitual operation of an office that attends to the poor and the seemingly banal details of daily life in a marginal neighborhood may not arrest one's attention in the same way as other potential empirical objects. Yet I hope to show that with regard to domination, the devil is in the details that can only be detected in these ostensibly dull universes. In order to cast light on the daily reproduction of political domination, I focus on the everyday interactions that take place between welfare clients and state agents, applicants for an ID and state officials, and shantytown dwellers and government bureaucrats. In these universes, much like in the world depicted in the classic film *Casablanca*, the "unfortunate ones" who lack money, influence, and connections are forced to endure "tortuous, roundabout" waiting periods. They are also subjected to all sort of minor indignities, amounting to a "ritual degradation of a pariah class" (Piven and Cloward 1971: 149). They endure the uncomfortable physical conditions of waiting; experience abrupt, unexplained changes in the system that exacerbate the uncertainty and arbitrariness pervading their lives; and are taught through these experiences that, in their dealings with the state, there is not much alternative other than to become a patient.

Kafka's *The Trial* calls attention to the arbitrariness and uncertainty that occur *during the course of waiting*, and therefore offers us another very helpful sensitizing viewpoint. The central character moves from initial detachment to full involvement in the process as he awaits his sentence. After having been slandered, Josef K. goes on with his life without disruption. As he states early in the story, "I'm completely detached from this whole affair." Yet as the book progresses, and as he progressively loses control, he is slowly inducted in the process and his concerns and anxiety begin to rise and take over his mind and body: "K. waited from day to day throughout the following week for further notification; he couldn't believe they had taken his waiver of interrogations literally, and when the expected notification had not arrived by Saturday evening, he took it as an implicit summons to appear again in the same building at the same time" (1998 [1946]: 54). The book wonderfully captures the protracted process of becoming ensnared in the web of the obscure and uncertain court proceedings. Halfway through the novel, K.'s initial cool detachment gradually becomes full investment: "The thought of his trial never left him now. . . . It was no longer a matter of accepting or rejecting the trial, he was in the midst of it and had to defend himself" (111–12). In the transition, the objective uncertainty (neither K. nor the reader know what he is being accused of, what the judiciary steps to follow are, and so on) becomes self-doubt: "Could he really rely so little on his own judgment already?" (137).

Beckett's Vladimir and Estragon are not alone in their waiting, and neither is K. During his progressive entrapment, he meets different characters (the uncle, the lawyer, the painter) that significantly influence his experience of the indeterminate trial. His subsequent encounters with these characters fill him with angst but also with hope. In what will turn out to be their last encounter, K. tells his lawyer: "You may have noticed during my first visit, when I came here with my uncle, that I wasn't particularly concerned about the trial . . ." But after engaging the lawyer, things begin to change: "I never had as many worries about the trial as I did from the moment you began to represent me. . . . I kept waiting expectantly for you to take action, but nothing was done" (187). His encounter with the painter highlights the unpredictability of the process but also the positive expectations generated during some his interactions: "If the judges could really be swayed as easily through personal contacts as the lawyer had suggested, then the painter's contacts with vain judges were particularly important and should by no means be underestimated. The painter would fit perfectly into the circle of helpers K. was gradually assembling about him" (151). His subjective investment in this process is therefore not an individual act but one that is carried out *in the company of others*, and this was one of the central analytical lessons I brought to the field. Others recurrently make "vain promises," "references to progress on the petition, to the improved mood of court officials, but also to the immense difficulties involved" (189), thereby collectively constructing the waiting as a *relational process*. We should thus pay particular attention to both horizontal and vertical interactions. There are both the exchanges that the destitute waiters establish among themselves and those with state agents who "in the name of a supposed familiarity with a powerful and worrying institution" (Bourdieu 2000: 230) blow hot and cold, alternatively troubling and reassuring the waiters. In this way, Kafka's character alerts us that waiting is both a *process* and a set of *power-laden relations*.

THE WHY IS IN THE HOW

The political scientist Rebecca Weitz-Shapiro's doctoral dissertation, "Choosing Clientelism" (2008), is an insightful, original study of why state officials decide to select patronage as a viable electoral strategy. It begins with the following scene:

Getting off the bus on the main road a short walk from the municipal building in the municipality of Campo Santo, in the province of Salta in Argentina, it is not difficult to find the social welfare area. It is prominently located near the main entrance of the municipality and, more importantly, identifiable by the sizable crowd of residents waiting to be attended. The crowd is made up mostly of women, many with small children, although one or two elderly are waiting, as well. . . . The type of requests they make vary widely: as I arrive, an elderly man is asking for help filling a prescription, while later in the morning a mother comes by to pick up a mattress she had recently requested so that her daughter could sleep in her own bed. Others have likely come to request they be added to the list of beneficiaries for a regular food distribution program or to inquire when the next disbursement for that program will take place. A sizable crowd also waits outside the mayor's office, located just down the hall from the social welfare area. (1–2)

During Weitz-Shapiro's dissertation defense, which I attended, one of her supervisors explicitly referred to this opening narrative. He also noted the many other descriptions of poor people's waiting contained in her work and then wondered out loud: "Why do they put up with this waiting?" The discussion suddenly turned away from the dissertation's main subject (the reasons why politicians "choose" clientelism) and briefly became a debate about the reasons why poor clients tolerate the long lines vividly described by the author. One of the other committee members knew I was the only person in the room who had conducted research on urban poverty, and thus directed the admittedly general (and probably rhetorical) question to me: "You've done research among the poor, why do you think they put up with that long wait?" Although I do not remember my exact words, I do recall feeling somewhat intimidated by the group of intelligent, well-known scholars at this highly prestigious university as well as somewhat surprised by the admitted absence of firsthand knowledge. I fumbled an answer along these lines: "Well, poor people in Argentina and elsewhere, have always been waiting . . . that's their life." It was not a very articulate, thoughtful answer, and both the question and my careless, off-the-cuff remark continued to bother me long after the dissertation defense was over. The exchange highlighted a modal but generally unknown experience among the poor and also directed the attention to the ways in which the destitute live under political domination. At the same time, it illustrated one of the ways in which the powerful exert their power: they make others wait. Barry Schwartz puts it succinctly: "Far from being a coincidental by product of power . . . control of time comes into view as one of its essential properties" (1974: 869).

Why do poor people comply with unbearably long and sometimes infinite waiting? This question is a version of another, which has been a central preoccupation among many a social scientist: How does domination work? Why do the subordinated yield to the wishes or desires of the dominant, who in this case tell them to wait? From Marx to Weber, from Gramsci and Althusser to Foucault and Bourdieu, numerous concepts have been deployed to address such perennial questions: dominant ideologies, legitimacy, hegemony, discipline, governmentality, ideological apparatus, and symbolic violence. Although I do not offer a review of these authors and concepts I will deploy some of their proposed thinking tools, which have been put to good use in empirical research elsewhere (Burawoy 1982; Gaventa 1980; Gilliom 2001; Scheper-Hughes 1994; Alford and Szanto 1996; Wacquant 2003a; Bourgois and Schonberg 2009), in order to understand and explain why poor people consent to extensive periods of waiting. The why is found not in factors or "variables" outside the very experience of waiting but in its inner dynamics. In other words, the why is in the how (Tilly 2006, 2008). Accordingly, my project in this book is to closely inspect the things poor people do, think, and feel while they endure such lengthy waits, and the many things they are explicitly and implicitly told to think and to do by those in power. The acquiescence of the subordinate is not something secured once and for all but is the result of a *process*, in which mystification plays a key role (Lukes 2004; Tilly 1997a). Poor people's actions, feelings, and thoughts while they wait for a welfare benefit or for a court ruling may look unimportant, but they are highly consequential for the production of compliance. These processes are thus an integral part of the daily and silent re-creation of political domination, which masks itself as an exercise of power and secures poor people's subjugation by constraining their use of time and by preventing conflict from arising.

TWO | Urban Relegation and Forms
of Regulating Poverty

Three decades of neoliberal economic policy have generated massive
dislocations and collective suffering in Argentina. Although many of
the economic changes brought about by the military dictatorship of
1976–1983 had neoliberal features, the main period of neoliberalization—as that truly political "vehicle for the restoration of class power"
(Harvey 2005; see also Peck and Tickell 2002)—took place in the early
1990s and had the following main characteristics: financial deregula-
tion, privatization, labor markets flexibility, and trade liberalization
(Teubal 2004; Cooney 2007).[1] During the first half of the 1990s, the
"swift and thorough" (Teubal 2004: 181) neoliberal experiment in Argentina generated high rates of economic growth (though decoupled
from employment generation) and monetary stability. The longer-
term result, though, was a second, deep wave of deindustrialization
(the first one took place during the military dictatorship) and its attendant deproletarianization, resulting in a "growing heterogeneous mass
of unemployed people without institutional protection from either
the state, the unions, or other organizations" (Villalón 2007: 140).
The economist Paul Cooney puts it this way: "[Since Menem became
president], there were major layoffs, totaling more than 110,000, as a
result of the privatizations that took place. Secondly, the decline in
manufacturing led to a reduction of over 369,000 jobs from 1991–
2001, a 33.9% loss in total manufacturing employment. As a result of
the two waves of deindustrialization, Argentina went from over 1.5
million manufacturing jobs in 1974 down to roughly 763 thousand
jobs in 2001, a loss of 50%" (2007: 23). The disappearance of formal

manufacturing jobs went hand in hand with the growth of informal employment. As Cooney further states: "Informal work in Buenos Aires and surroundings (*Gran Buenos Aires*) grew to reach 38% of all employment by 1999, and such jobs are estimated to have incomes 45% lower than formal employment" (24). Thus, from the early 1990s until the early 2000s the impoverishment of the middle- and low-income sectors was driven by the disappearance of formal work and an explosion in unemployment levels. In this, the Argentine experience with neoliberalism, despite being "extreme" (Teubal 2004), was unexceptional; as elsewhere it has resulted in "a fall in popular consumption, a deterioration of social conditions, a rise in poverty, immiseration and insecurity, heightened inequalities, social polarization, and resultant political conflict" (Robinson 2008: 20). The most dramatic physical manifestation of this generalized degradation in the lives of the dispossessed is found in the explosive growth of the population living in informal settlements, both *villas* (shantytowns) and *asentamientos* (squatter settlements).

The authors María Cristina Cravino, Juan Pablo del Río, and Juan Ignacio Duarte provide a thorough description of the rapid increase in "informal settlements" in the metropolitan area of Buenos Aires, which is comprised of the city of Buenos Aires and the twenty-four bordering districts known as Conurbano Bonaerense.[2] According to these authors, as of 2006 there were 819 informal settlements—363 shantytowns, 429 squatter settlements, and 27 unspecified urban forms—with approximately 1 million residents. This represents 10.1 percent of the total population of the metropolitan area of Buenos Aires. This figure is almost double what it was in 1991 (5.2 percent) and much larger than it was in 1981 (4.3 percent) (2008: 14).

Between 1981 and 2006, the total population in the Conurbano Bonaerense grew by 35 percent, while the population in shantytowns and squatter settlements in the same region increased by 220 percent. If we look at the figures since the economic collapse of 2001, we see that most of the total population growth took place in informal settlements. Between 2001 and 2006, for every 100 new residents in the Conurbano, 60 are found in informal settlements, compared to 10 for every 100 between 1981 and 1991 and 26 for every 100 between 1991 and 2001 (Cravino et al. 2008: 13).[3]

The proliferation of shantytowns and squatter settlements is a concrete geographical expression of the fragmentation of Buenos Aires's metropolitan space, which in turn reflects and reinforces growing levels of social inequality (Catenazzi and Lombardo 2003). During the last three decades, there has been a steady widening of the distribution of income in the country as a whole and therefore a mounting disparity between Argentines. As Ricardo Aronskind summarizes: "21.5% of the population was poor in 1991, 27% at the end of 2000. Indigents were 3% of the population in 1991 and 7% in 2000. At the beginnings of the 1990s there were 1.6 million unemployed, at the end of 2000 there are 4 million unemployed" (2001: 18). If we take recent figures available from the National Institute of Statistics (INDEC), the rising poverty rates become quite evident. In 1986, 9.1 percent of households and 12.7 percent of people lived below the poverty line in Greater Buenos Aires. In 2002, these figures were 37.7 percent and 49.7 percent, respectively. In other words, whereas a little more than one in ten *bonaerenses* was poor twenty years ago, at the dawn of the new century one in two is living below the poverty line. With respect to inequality, one figure should suffice: the Gini coefficient went from .36 in 1974 to .51 in 2000 (Altimir et al. 2002: 54).

Since 2003, however, poverty rates seem to be declining.[4] The GDP has been growing at an annual rate of 9 percent and unemployment and poverty rates have decreased to the mid-1990s levels. And yet, 34 percent of the total population lives below the poverty line, and 12 percent subsists under the indigence line (Salvia 2007: 28). Even after the economic recovery that began in 2003, poor people's material and symbolic conditions were deeply affected by the sustained decline of income levels in the lower rungs of the job market and the growth of informal employment.

Despite these more positive trends, economic and social disparities have become inscribed in urban space. Gated *barrios privados* (suburban communities that Pedro Pírez refers to as "corridors of modernity and wealth" [2001: 3]) have been mounting alongside enclaves of dep-

rivation (Svampa 2001). These barrios privados, compared to the villas
and new asentamientos, now encapsulate the growing extremes of poverty and wealth that characterize contemporary Argentina. In other
words, to borrow an expression from Patrick Heller and Peter Evans,
villas and barrios privados "showcase the most durable and disturbing
forms of contemporary inequality" (2010: 433). The following is a
selection of excerpts written by a journalist who captures this class
divide in a simple, illuminating, way:

Florencia Tedin grew up wealthy, but says she never felt any distinction between her prospects and those of her cleaning lady's children.

For years, it was a common Argentine assumption that a taxi driver's son
could become a lawyer, the plumber's daughter a psychoanalyst.

But not any more. On a recent day, Ms. Tedin looks at the woman caring
for her four small children in their rambling home in a gated community
outside Buenos Aires and shakes her head sadly. Today, she says, maids'
children will be maids.

The gap between rich and poor has slowly expanded over the decades in
a society that has always thought of itself as Latin America's model for egali-
tarianism. . . .

While unemployment has halved, from around 20 percent at the height of
the (2001) crisis, half of all jobs are in the informal sector. Few provide
benefits, protection, or true prospects for mobility . . .

The income divide is apparent just beyond the gates Ms. Tedin must pass
to access her driveway. Her family relocated to this gated community, where
100 families live on 100 plots of land, for security, says Tedin, who grew up in
the same area, but in the center of town.

Known as "countries," they were once the weekend getaways for the urban elite, but now more and more Buenos Aires residents are making them
their permanent homes.

Some communities are massive mini-cities with schools, churches, and
shopping centers. "It's a little bit like the 'Truman Show,'" says Tedin, whose
manicured lawn looks onto an artificial lake.

"If the country becomes secure again, I'd like to live outside," she says.

Only a few blocks away, on the main road, Nieve Barrio lives in a simple concrete home. Many of her neighborhood's streets are unpaved dirt alleys that become giant puddles when it rains. Most residents are domestic workers like Ms. Barrio, or bricklayers and gardeners, and many work in the gated communities nearby. Barrio also mends clothes on the side.

Barrio says she raised six children as a single mother on a maid's salary, but that is no longer possible today.[5]

In the following section I provide an ethnographic portrait of how the relegation of impoverished and marginalized individuals created by the aforementioned structural transformation of the Argentine economy looks like at the ground level. What follows should be read as a rough sketch of what we could call a "relegated space"—one inhabited by masses of informal workers and unemployed individuals who barely make ends meet, and characterized by crumbling infrastructure, by dysfunctional institutions, and by all sorts of environmental hazards that the different levels of the state are unwilling or incapable of preventing or reducing.

RELEGATION IN REAL TIME AND SPACE

> Relegate: To consign (a person or thing) to some unimportant or obscure position, or to a particular role, esp. one of inferiority.
> —*Oxford English Dictionary*

The following series of fieldnotes present a brief slice of the daily life among the destitute. They were taken by Flavia Bellomi, an elementary school teacher who was once an aspiring anthropologist and is now my research collaborator.[6] The fieldnotes, written between May and August 2009, intend to simultaneously capture Bellomi's daily activities as an elementary school teacher in two schools adjacent to a newer squatter settlement in one of the poorest districts of metropolitan Buenos Aires and the diverse risks to which poor children are exposed in their schools and in their neighborhoods. Her notes vividly illustrate that poor people's physical integrity is constantly assaulted by both interpersonal violence and by the material living conditions both inside and outside of the school where they live, eat, play, and learn. Dozens of pages of Bellomi's diary attest to the sad and simple fact that children in Buenos Aires's "neighborhoods of relegation" (Wacquant 2009) attend relegated schools that warehouse future generations while barely acting as bulwarks against the dangers of daily life.

May 5: During lunchtime, a student from third grade shows his plate to the teacher. There's a dead (and cooked) cockroach. We told the school principal. The students kept eating as usual.

May 6: As I am entering the school building, Luis's mother comes to talk to me. Luis has not been in school for at least a month. She tells me they've been living in the street, sleeping in a kind of storage space. They were allowed to stay there until 5 AM. Then they would start scavenging the streets and asking for food in restaurants and bars. They are now renting a house in a nearby barrio. They are all from the province of Formosa. . . . She begins to cry as she tells me her story. She tells me that she was very scared while sleeping on the streets. She is worried for Luis: she doesn't want him to miss more classes. Luis's face is full of scars.

At 9 AM my students had PE. One of them, Fernanda, fell and banged her head. We call the emergency service and, luckily, they came quickly. Since Fernanda began to vomit, we had to take her to the local hospital. We called ahead because there's usually no pediatrician there.

Almost every single day my students ask me if we are going to have class tomorrow [because of strikes and classes cancelled due to problems in the building, children had an average of three school days per week].

May 7: In class, my students (third grade) tell me that there are new residents in the nearby squatter settlement (where most of them live) and that they have brought in drugs. Every night, they tell me, there are shootouts. They also say that there are now many more drugs around.

May 11: Today, the smell from the purifying plant (located adjacent to the school) is unbearable. We can't open the window of the classroom because we are right in front of it. During lunchtime, the kids don't want to eat. They tell me: "It's really disgusting to eat with this odor." The plant has been malfunctioning for the last seventeen years.

May, 15: In order to go to the cafeteria to have breakfast, we now need to go through the outside patio because the covered patio is closed. The roof there is about to fall off.

May 15: A friend of mine who teaches at a nearby school tells me classes had to be cancelled there because dead rats were found in the water tank. Dozens of teachers and students were suffering gastroenteritis. Since last year, that same school does not have a working gas connection—thus, no heating; thus, no kid can drink anything hot.

May 18: Luis was very sleepy today. He went to bed at 3 AM because he went back to scavenging with his family. He reminded me of another student I had in Villa Fiorito a couple of years ago. One day he came with his hand bitten by a rat. Apparently, he was eating and he fell asleep and the rat took his food [and bit his hand in the attempt].

June 3: A girl from fourth grade came to school with a serious injury in her abdomen. She had a fight with her sister who threw a glass at her. She went to the local hospital but there were no supplies to stitch up her injury. So, she went back home and then came to school. We had to call her mom to pick her up.

June 9: A student's mother came to see me. Her son, Manuel, has been absent for many days. She tells me that Manuel is full of pimples—just like her eight other children . . . They live along the [highly contaminated] banks of [a dead river known as] the Riachuelo.

August 3: I arrive in school at 7:30 AM and the principal tells me that part of the ceiling in the main area of the school fell off. This part of the school is now closed. The other area which was closed months ago has not yet been repaired.

Some of the excerpts above reveal the daily denial of adequate infrastructure and routine absence of protection from environmental hazards and risks that I analyzed elsewhere (Auyero and Swistun 2009). Other excerpts show that, on a daily basis, Bellomi's students are exposed to diverse kinds of violence. They witness shootings, murders, and episodes of sexual and domestic violence from an early age. During the eighteen months that Bellomi recorded in her field diary not a week went by without one or more of them (whose ages range from seven to thirteen) describing one or more episodes involving one or more forms of violence. This rampant violence is, in my view, *new*. Fifteen years ago I conducted eight months of fieldwork in a nearby shantytown and described what at the time, borrowing from Loïc Wacquant's analysis of the "hyper-ghetto" (1995, 1998) and Philippe Bourgois's examination of crack dealing in the inner-city (2003 [1995]), I defined as the depacification of daily life in the hyper-shantytown (Auyero 2000). Residents of the shantytown, knowing that at the time of my fieldwork I was living in New York, and drawing upon global stereotypes of localized violence, asked me if their neighborhood was "just like the Bronx" (Auyero 1999). Back then residents quite often experienced muggings at night or in the early hours of the morning when they were heading to work. And they complained about the occasional shooting and the increasing presence of drugs. But violence was confined to a specific group of known perpetrators (small-scale drug dealers who, though a minority, managed to set the tone of public life in the barrio) and to certain "no-go" areas of the neighborhood. The violence I examined back then pales in comparison to what residents are experiencing these days. Official data for the province of Buenos Aires show a doubling of crime rates between 1995 (the year of my fieldwork) and 2008 (from 1,114 to 2,010 criminal episodes per 100,000 residents; and from 206 to 535 crimes against persons per 100,000 residents). Yet these numbers scarcely do justice to the violence that now suffuses everyday life in the neighborhood—keeping residents on edge, "watching out" constantly—as people frequently warn each other, "Hay que tener cuidado" (You have to be careful). It is beyond the scope of this book to attempt to explain the increase of daily violence that is currently ravaging the daily life of the urban poor.[7] I should note, however, that this new violence is undoubtedly related to the increasing reliance of economically marginalized and vulnerable people on the destructive drug trade. The drug economy is, numerous studies have shown (for the United States, see Bourgois 2003; for Argentina, see Alarcón 2009) a double-edged sword: it sustains poor communities as it simultaneously tears them apart. But this is only part of the causal story that is behind the intensification of daily violence. The great neoliberal transformation, outlined above, and state actions (and inactions) are also part of the "whys" of violence (Portes and Roberts 2005). The growth of daily violence is then an effect of a complex causal chain whose origin lies in the economy (deproletarianization, informalization, expansion of drug trade, general degradation in living conditions, increasing social isolation) and in the state (the lack of institutions that address seriously and systematically sexual violence; the state's losing monopoly over legitimate state violence; increasing punitive regulation of poverty; and the low-intensity citizenship for the urban poor that translates into the routine denial and violation of rights).

The great neoliberal transformation has triggered diverse forms of unruly behavior among the destitute that take the shape of street protests, land squatting, and diverse forms of delinquency. Poor people's unrest has been met in turn by fierce actions from the state apparatus. The visible iron fist of the Argentine state has been quite busy during the last two decades. It has openly repressed protests organized by the unemployed, persistently criminalized contentious collective action, dramatically increased the prison population, engaged in high levels of police violence against poor youth, deployed military-style forces such as the National Guard to provide "safety" inside (but in actuality to occupy and rein in) certain destitute and highly stigmatized urban areas, and sharply increased the number of evictions carried out by state agents on private and public property (CELS 2003, 2009; Brinks 2008a, 2008b).

But the visible fist has not acted alone. Other forms of repression (what I call "clandestine kicks") as well as less visible forms of power have also been active in the state's attempt both to control poor people's actions and to manufacture their acquiescence. In order to understand the routine political production of poor people's subordination, in the sections following I flesh out the workings of fists and kicks as incarnations of state-generated collective violence. What Charles Tilly calls "violence specialists"—that is, actors who specialize in "inflict-ing physical damage such as police, soldiers, guards, thugs, and gangs" (2003: 35)—play a key, though sometimes not quite discernible, role in the origins and the course of state-employed violence. Another way in which the state seeks to achieve poor people's submission is what I call "invisible tentacles." This is power exercised by minor state bureau-crats working for usually underfunded welfare agencies, and thus it is mostly devoid of physical violence. In this chapter I capture in sche-matic form the political production of patients of the state and situate this production within a larger menu of poverty-regulation strategies. The chapters that follow will then empirically substantiate this theo-retical argument.

In the sections following I outline these forms of regulating of pov-erty as "vehicles for the political production of reality and for the oversight of deprived and defamed social categories and their reserved territories" (Wacquant 2009: 304).[8] I argue by way of demonstration that for a better understanding of the relationship between poor peo-ple's domination and the politics of collective violence, we should pay attention to the *simultaneous operation of these three forces (fists, kicks, and tentacles) in the daily life of the destitute*. This allows us to better integrate violence into the study of popular politics, something that most political analysis neglects (Tilly 2003), and to cast light on the productive—as opposed to merely repressive—nature of state power (Foucault 1979; Wacquant 2009).

In drawing upon primary and secondary sources, including past and present ethnographic fieldwork, investigative reporters' accounts, and human rights reports, I depict in detail poor peoples' various encoun-ters with the state. Collectively, these accounts from varied sources present a unified landscape, whether they describe the dwellers of hous-ing projects being besieged by the National Guard, squatters being evicted by policemen and paramilitary forces, or clients endlessly wait-ing at the state welfare office. This landscape is the modal encounter between the dispossessed and the state, characterized by the routine truncation or utter denial of the most elementary forms of citizenship.

To foreshadow some of the substantive points of this chapter, I begin with one individual's story, which in actuality is a composite created out of several stories I heard in the field. This story encapsulates multiple forms of power that poor people experience in their daily encounters with the state. It also serves as a roadmap for the exposition that follows: it moves from a description of overt forms of state coercion to a dissection of a less forceful but equally relevant form of domination. In sum, my main argument here is that state power, whether it is overt or covert violence or exhibits more "gentle" forms, not only punishes the poor but also attempts to discipline them, producing what I call "patients of the state." The nitty-gritty details of this manufacturing will be the subject of the chapters that follow, and as they progress I will occasionally come back to Jessica's seemingly unremarkable but quite illustrative story.

Jessica, born and raised in Argentina, is nineteen years old. We met her at the welfare office in the city of Buenos Aires. She came to renew her housing subsidy. She has been waiting for four hours and, like most of the people we talked to in the office during our fieldwork, she does not know if and when she will receive the benefit. "You come here and you don't know at what time you'll leave." As we are speaking with her, a state agent tells her, from the counter and in a very teacher-like manner, "stay seated." She turns to us and says: "If they are in a good mood, they treat you well."

Like many other recipients of the housing subsidy, Jessica first heard about it from a social worker who was present when state officials and policemen were evicting her and fifteen other families with children ("we were all women, with children in tow") from her room of "wood and metal shingles" in a squatter settlement. She still remembers the day of the eviction as a highly traumatic experience—"there were these guys, throwing all our stuff into garbage trucks."

Jessica thinks the welfare benefit is an "aid because with the scavenging, I can't pay for a room. These days, it costs at least $450 a month (roughly US$110), and with the scavenging I collect for the day to day, I can't pay the rent with it." If she is lucky, the subsidy will cover six months of rent in a run-down hotel in the city. After those six months, she will be homeless; the subsidy cannot be renewed.

Echoing what we heard countless times, Jessica says that obtaining the benefit takes "a long time . . . you never know when they will pay you." And like many others, she conceives of the waiting time as an indicator of the clients' perseverance and thus of their "real need." If you "really need," she and others believe, "you will wait for a long time," you will "keep coming," and you will show state agents you are worthy of aid. This is how she puts it: "You have to wait, wait, and wait. . . . They will not give it to you until you come here three, four, five, ten times, to check, to talk, to ask, with this one or with the other one . . ."

Like many people we talked to, Jessica compares this long and uncertain wait to that of the public hospital; and, in a statement that captures one prominent way in which poor people relate to the state, she adds: "Here and in the hospital, they tell you the same thing, 'sit down and wait' . . . and (what do you do?), you sit down and wait. And if you have some money, you buy a soda and a sandwich" [my emphasis].

The progression of Jessica's story corresponds to the narrative sequence of the remainder of this chapter. I first examine the visible fists (the forceful eviction), then depict clandestine kicks (the actions of "the guys," who, as we will see, are thugs working for the state), and finish with a sketch of the workings of even less visible forms of power ("sit down and wait"). For both narrative and analytic purposes, this chapter separates these forces. We should not forget, however, that they are deeply intertwined in the daily encounters between the urban poor and the state.

The contemporary gargantuan expansion of the prison system in the United States and Europe and the concentration of this massive growth among specific racial and ethnic groups are the subjects of much research in the social sciences (e.g., Garland 2006; Western 2006; Wacquant 2009). Recently, however, scholarship has also begun to pay sustained and systematic attention to the ways in which this unprecedented mass incarceration is affecting everyday life in poor communities (Goffman 2009; Comfort 2008). This chapter adds to this new literature in two ways: first, it presents findings from the little-known case of contemporary Argentina on the manifold ways in which the neoliberal state has coaxed the urban poor into compliance; and second, it extends the forms of the regulation of mass misery from incarceration and repression to less overt and more subtle kinds of power.

VISIBLE FISTS

I want to make two disclaimers here at the outset of my discussion of visible fists. First, the hardening of state power against poor people in the form of violence, imprisonment, evictions, and territorial control does not obey a deliberate plan designed by authorities, but rather is an "objective convergence of a welter of disparate public policies" (Wacquant 2009: 29). In this sense, the image of a fist can be misleading. There is neither a deliberate plan nor a single, monolithic agent driving the fist against the poor; rather, it is a series of processes that coalesce around the management of their conduct. Second, when dealing with the subaltern, state agents do not always carry out their business in broad daylight. As we will see in the case of evictions undertaken in the city of Buenos Aires, the public dimension of the democratic state sometimes vanishes when interacting with marginal populations. In such situations, the state's operation instead resembles the covert workings of a dictatorial state that has terrifying resonances in Argentine history (O'Donnell 1993; Brinks 2008a, 2008b). The image of clandestine kicks seeks to capture this other form of state action.

Protest, repression and criminalization. Since the return of democracy in 1983, the repression of poor peoples' social movements by the state has ebbed and flowed. During the second half of the 1990s and early 2000s, state violence reached a brutal extreme with the repression of unemployed protesters (known as *piqueteros*) and the street demonstrations of December 2001 (Giarracca 2001; Svampa and Pereyra 2003). Security agents routinely made informal use of lethal force to quell massive protest, thus implicating the Argentine state in serious human rights violations. Between December 1999 and June 2002, twenty-two people were killed by state forces in public protests and hundreds were seriously injured (CELS 2003). Although state violence against piqueteros has decreased since 2003, the judicial criminalization of protest persists (CELS 2009). In the last decade, thousands of protesters have been prosecuted by the state. The "tremendous coercive power deployed against those accused in a penal process" has thus been used "by the administration of justice as an authentic tool to subjugate activists" (CELS 2003: 24; see also CELS 2009).

Police violence. According to Daniel Brinks (2008a: 12), twenty-five years of democracy has had "a noticeably democratizing impact on the written laws and constitutions of Latin America." He continues by stating:

> If the laws described the practice, Latin America would be approaching an egalitarian democratic utopia, and yet the de facto world of discrimination and rights violations continues to outdistance the de jure world of equal rights for all. *Police violence* is one of the places where the reality does not live up to the promise of democracy. Many countries, even or especially those with a legacy of authoritarian repression, have become political democracies but continue to violate individual rights. These countries no longer target political opponents, but their police continue to torture and kill on a large scale *in the interest of social order.* (Brinks 2008a: 12; my emphasis)

Among Latin American countries, Argentina (along with Brazil) stands out. The country's security forces rely habitually on deadly violence as a means to control crime (Daroqui et al. 2009). The human rights report published annually by the Centro de Estudios Legales y Sociales (CELS) puts it this way: "The high levels of violence . . . the abusive use of force, the extrajudicial executions of those suspected of a crime, the arbitrary detentions, the torture and the physical abuse, the fabrication of criminal cases and the false imputations, still are extended phenomena in Argentina" (CELS 2009: 11). Between 1995 and 2000, Buenos Aires "averaged a per capita rate of police homicides (almost 2 per hundred thousand) . . . that was just as high as the [noticeably violent] Sao Paulo" (Brinks 2008a: 12). This unabated and usually unpunished police violence is needless to say not democratic. It targets the urban poor and, among them, the youth living in shanty-towns, housing projects, and squatter settlements (CELS 2009; Daroqui et al. 2009).

Prison growth. Another facet of the state's visible fist is the runaway growth of the prison population. Like many advanced societies, Argentina has seen a "spectacular swelling of the population behind bars" (Wacquant 2009: xiii). Although there is a remarkable difference in the rates of incarceration between Argentina and the United States (183.5 convicts per 100,000 residents in 2007 versus 760 per 100,000 in the United States), both countries have witnessed this prison expansion during the last two decades. In the United States, the imprisonment rate went from 138 convicts per 100,000 residents in 1980 to 478 per 100,000 in 2000 (Wacquant 2009: 117). Since the return of democracy, Argentina has seen an almost fourfold increase (398 percent) in the population of federal prisons. In Buenos Aires, for example, there were 14,292 persons in state jails and prisons in 1997; a decade later, the incarcerated population had almost doubled to 27,614 (CELS 2009). At the time of this writing, there are 30,194 persons behind bars (CELS 2010; Verbitsky 2010). Of these inmates 68 percent do not have a firm judicial sentence (i.e., they are imprisoned under pretrial detention), and 30 percent of them will be declared innocent when their cases close (according to the statistics produced by the state government). In the best documented case, that of the province of Buenos Aires, this phenomenal increase is related neither to demographic growth (less than 10 percent) nor to crime intensification. Between 1990 and 2007, the crime rate increased by 64 percent (CELS 2010; Verbitsky 2010); between 1994 and 2009, the incarceration rate increased by 200 percent—from 95 per 100,000 residents to 194 per 100,000 residents (see fig. 1).[9] Of those behind bars in the province of

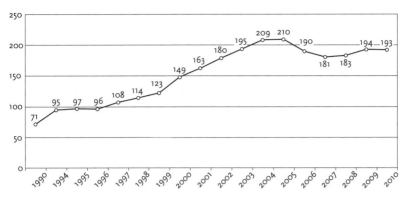

1 Prisonization rates (per 100,000 residents) in the province of Buenos Aires. Centro de Estudios Legales y Sociales (CELS), based on data from the Servicio Penitenciario Bonaerense, the Ministerio de Justicia y Seguridad de la Provincia de Buenos Aires, and the Instituto Nacional de Estadísticas y Censos (INDEC).

Buenos Aires, 78 percent are between eighteen and forty-four years old (96 percent of them are men) and the overwhelming majority comes from the most dispossessed urban groups: 7 percent of those incarcerated have never attended an educational institution, 23 percent did not finish elementary school, 53 percent have only finished elementary school, and 13 percent drop out of high school.[10] At the time of the arrest, 51 percent were unemployed and 27 percent were part-time workers.

The Centro de Estudios Legales y Sociales has publicly denounced the appalling living conditions inside the overcrowded Argentine prisons and the systematic violation of inmates' rights.[11] The following statement about Latin American prisons in general applies exactly to the case of Argentina: "Killings, overcrowding, disease, torture, hunger, corruption, and the abuse of due process that occur under the twenty-four-hour watch of the state belie the principles underlying contemporary Latin American democracy" (Ungar and Magaloni 2009: 223; see also Müller 2012).

It is beyond the scope of this work to present a full comparison between imprisonment in the advanced north and the underdeveloped south. Nevertheless, in both cases "incarceration rates serve to physically neutralize and warehouse the supernumerary fractions of the working class and in particular the dispossessed members of the stigmatized groups" (Wacquant 2009: xvi). As the CELS report states, the prison is used as a "generalized state response to social conflicts and claims" (2009: 279)—the prison is thus used as an instrument to regulate poverty.

Military occupation. Another particularly illustrative case of state control over the behavior of the urban poor has been the occupation of entire neighborhoods by the National Guard (Gendarmería Nacional) in what amounts to veritable territorial sieges. The National Guard is a security force with military origins that is dependent on the Ministry of Justice, Security and Human Rights of the Argentine Nation. The gendarmes now enforce law and order in the infamous neighborhoods of La Cava and Carlos Gardel in Buenos Aires (*Revista Mu*, 2008). Yet it is in the barrio Ejército de los Andes, also commonly known as Fuerte Apache, that the national guardsmen have achieved national notoriety. Approximately 35,000 people live in the barrio's 3,777 apartments. The neighborhood is located in Ciudadela and is a few blocks from General Paz, which is the highway that divides Greater Buenos Aires—a metropolitan area that compromises twenty-four municipal districts—from the central city. *Los tortugas ninja* (ninja turtles), as the national guardsmen are locally known, have been an occupying force in this neighborhood since November 14, 2003, and their stated mission is "improving security."

The following is a selection of excerpts written by the journalist Cristian Alarcón after the assassination of a guardsman in the neighborhood. The full story uncovers retaliation as a factor in the murder and exposes the relational and honorific character of the violence, which is portrayed as meaningless by the media and authorities. The selected passages illustrate vividly how poor people live with the daily violence exerted by state agents:

"I was going to study, almost two weeks ago. We had been eating home-made bread," says P., 20 years old, unemployed since they fired him from his job as a food distributor. "Five or six guardsmen came then, there are never fewer than five or six, with batons to hit [us with]. They have helmets, and armor, and look like Ninja Turtles. They tell you: 'Don't look at me. Look down. Drop to the floor. Don't look at me idiot, and then they take out everything you have in your pockets. If there is money, somewhere, depending on the guardsman, he keeps it. If not, they take the drugs and give you everything else back."

Alarcón points out that P's story is quite typical. Guards routinely order poor youngsters "not to look" at them, and "kick their heels with cruelty and verbally denigrate them." His report continues: "In each [entrance to the neighborhood] there is a security post; in each post, between three and five uniformed men. Those who guard do not look like those that walk in the neighborhood; they wear military clothes and carry heavy weapons. After ten o'clock . . . the Special Forces come out, or the so-called *cascudos* (the 'helmeted') . . . . The tension with the guardsmen can be felt in the darkness on Friday night. Between the dirty walls of one of the buildings, the light of a flashlight moves as if looking for something. It looks like one of those huge lights they turn on in jails when someone escapes. One can distinguish the silhouettes of the Ninja Turtles forming a troop of six . . . The guardsmen advance with their mouths closed and long rifles in hand. Like that, with signals, without saying a word, they order the young men they encounter to get against the wall. They make them put their hands up, open their legs and proceed to pat them down."[12]

Evictions. During the 1990s Buenos Aires experienced "a profound transformation of the built environment. Local effects of globalization seem to generate [the] expulsion of low-income sectors from areas of the city that are currently required by corporate agents for development and investment. These trends enhance urban segregation" (Procupez and Rodriguez 2001: 216). Market forces have not acted alone in reshaping the megacity's social geography. State-mandated evictions from illegally occupied residences and from public spaces have sky-rocketed since the beginning of the decade, especially in the city of Buenos Aires. This is due to the rapid increase in real estate prices since 2001, increasing gentrification in selected areas of the city, and changes in the judiciary that shorten the civil judicial process. When the current mayor of Buenos Aires took office, there were squatters and homeless individuals living in approximately 160 public spaces, mostly parks and plazas; in less than a year, the government "cleaned" almost 100 of them (*Perfil*, November 16, 2008). Evictions from private and state-owned buildings also quickly increased. In 2006, thirty-four people per day were evicted; a year later, seventy-six people a day were removed from the places where they were living (*Clarín*, June 2004, 2007). By the end of 2007, a total of 6,700 families had been evicted in the city of Buenos Aires (*Clarín*, September 7, 2007). According to the city government, there has been a 300 percent increase in evictions during 2007 (CELS 2009: 322). During 2008, evictions proceeded at an even faster pace: one eviction was ordered by the judiciary per day. In denying their speed but acknowledging their occurrence, the city government chief of staff put it this way: "*Slowly, and silently*, evictions are being carried out" (*Página12*, May 4, 2009; my emphasis).[13]

The State Can't Wait: Express Evictions

Belying the statement made by city government chief of staff regarding the pace of evictions, in the last two years the city administration has developed a new eviction protocol: Evictions are now carried out without the need to prove that a crime has been committed and without a hearing prior to the eviction procedure. According to a report prepared by the city ombudsman office based on a sample of 240 cases (randomly selected from the 1,169 judicial cases of "illegal occupation" initiated during 2009), 78% of those evicted could not count on a lawyer to defend themselves.[14]

Officials of the state program Buenos Aires Presente (BAP) deal with those recently evicted on a daily basis. They are usually present during

the evictions to offer shelter or a housing subsidy, and they also patrol
the streets in search for the homeless. In a dozen personal interviews,
all of them noted an important increase in the number of evictions
during the first year of the current city administration, which was
reflected in the number of "cases" they began to process. As one of
them puts it: "We have a lot of work now, with all the evictions."

Blanca, who stays with friends while awaiting a resolution on the
housing subsidy she applied for months ago, told us that she found out
about the welfare office "from a man at the ministry who referred us to
this office." When we asked her where she and this official met, her
response summarized the typical process: they met the day of the eviction. Those evicted are given the first installment of the housing subsidy and are then asked to go to the welfare office so that they can
process the paperwork to formally apply for it. At the office, they
oftentimes find out that they do not qualify because, as a BAP official
admits, sometimes during evictions "subsidies are given out without
such requirements in mind."

The number of people living in the streets doubled in less than a
year in 2009, from roughly one thousand to two thousand individuals
sleeping in the streets on any given night (*Página12*, May 4, 2009). As
the city government rolls out its punitive arm with rapidly increasing
evictions, it simultaneously withdraws its welfare hand. The budget of
the Instituto de Vivienda de la Ciudad (the agency in charge of state-
funded housing) decreased fourfold during the same period, from 500
million pesos to 120 million pesos. The following dialogues at the
welfare office illustrate the precarious housing situation of thousands
of residents of Buenos Aires, characterized by more evictions and
fewer, more expensive, more restrictive, and sometimes illegal transitory residences for the city poor.

Claudia rents an overpriced (US$300 per month) family room in a hotel in
downtown, with no private bathroom or kitchen. Why so expensive, we ask.
"I don't know, eh, I believe that it's good because everything is like that, I
looked around before renting this. Moreover because of the baby they don't
accept you in many places, and when they see you with one they charge

more." Almost every person who is living in a hotel told us that children are indeed an impediment to obtaining a room. As Cebelina puts it: "With kids it's harder. They don't want to rent to you with kids . . . they say that they damage the room." Cebelina is living in a hotel. Luckily for her they haven't collected [rent] for four months because the place has an eviction order. The landlord, whom Cebelina never met, "hasn't showed up during all of this time."

CLANDESTINE KICKS

"Come on, wake up, let's go!" The screams woke Maria up at dawn. Three men, dressed in black hooded sweatshirts, were tearing down her shack located below the highway.

"Come on! What's going on with you? Up! Or do you want me to bring the gang?" María crawled on the dirt floor, her eight-month pregnant belly hanging, facing down. The only thing she could see were the military-style pants and the sneakers that were kicking everything she had. A few meters away, a camouflaged garbage truck was waiting, engine on. The men threw her mattresses, her blankets, and three bags full of plastic bottles and cardboard into the truck.

Suddenly, there were noises of an ongoing fight. María's son grabbed a cart, his hands hard like iron claws.

"Let it go, little piece of shit [*pendejo de mierda*]!" the hooded man shouted at him and grabbed the cart, brusquely pushing the kid aside. In desperation, María ran toward her son. She arrived at the scene just in time to get a blow from a stick that sent her to the hospital with hemorrhages.

The *patota* [gang] got into the unidentified car [no plates] . . . From the floor, María was able to read the words in one of the men's caps: UCEP.[15]

Evictions are mandated by the state and are usually carried out with police assistance. Yet during the last two administrations, the city government has also deployed a special force whose task is to intimidate and then violently remove *intrusos* (intruders, unlawful tenants) from parks, plazas, streets, lots below highways, and city buildings. In 2009 a group of twenty to thirty "corpulent and unfriendly looking men"

(*Perfil*, November 16, 2008) was officially named the Unidad de Control del Espacio Público (UCEP). All of the UCEP members are state employees. Before the current administration, under "progressive" and self-identified center-left governments, the group was known informally as "the sharks." The press has documented dozens of violent evictions involving these enforcers. They usually conduct them at night, using methods that sadly resemble those used by military authorities during the last dictatorship to "clean up" the city of shantytown dwellers (Oszlak 1991; *Perfil*, November 16, 2008; *Página12*, May 4, 2009; *Página12*, April 12, 2009; *Notife*, August 3, 2009). As current officials from BAP acknowledge in personal interviews: "Yes, we know about the UCEP. It's a task force [*un grupo de tareas*] with characteristics that are similar to those deployed during the last military dictatorship." "They are members of a government program that gives people hell . . . a [homeless] woman I assist had her wheelchair compacted by the garbage truck they use!"

Since both groups (UCEP and BAP) deal with the homeless population, agents at the latter have reason to be concerned. In personal interviews, one of the program coordinators expressed his suspicions regarding the reports they write as part of their job, which record the locations of the homeless among other things: "I don't really know where our reports go. We write a social report, with basic data about people living on the street. Those reports might end up in the hands of UCEP. These aren't crazy suspicions!" This official is not alone in his misgivings. The CELS describes the UCEP as a "gang that counted on information collected by the BAP." And a psychologist interviewed by the press after resigning from the BAP told a similar story. Simultaneously highlighting the differentiated nature of the state and the practical complications of this differentiation, this psychologist asserts: "[When a homeless person told me that he was assaulted or threatened by the UCEP] it was very difficult, because with my BAP uniform, I felt that I was there in the name of the state and the city government, representing the very same policy carried out by the UCEP" (*Página12*, November 15, 2009).

When asked about their "cleaning" procedures, UCEP members assured journalists "that they are peaceful but that, on occasion, they have to show their teeth: 'One day an intruder didn't want to leave and we had to put a garbage truck in front of him and told him that we would throw all his stuff in there. He understood'" (*Perfil*, November 16, 2008).

Government officials and the "sharks" themselves say that all they do is "make people [intruders] comply [with the law]"; they seek to "clean up the public spaces from intruders, in the name of the law" (*Perfil*, November 16, 2008). What they do not admit is that they do so by unlawfully employing outright violence, causing physical harm to destitute city residents and destroying their few belongings. A joint report based on witnesses' accounts, carried out by the city ombudsman office, the Centro de Estudios Legales y Sociales, and the Defensoría Oficial de la Justicia Porteña, reconstructs a series of evictions and unambiguously describes the UCEP "as a para-police force that seeks to threaten, stigmatize, repress, and expel from the city the most vulnerable persons" (*Página12*, October 22, 2009).

The UCEP enforcers, true "violence specialists" (Tilly 2003), are the final and more recent incarnation of the state's clandestine kicks. They express the continuing operation of what in previous work I called the "gray zone" of state power (Auyero 2007): the informal, clandestine links between established powerholders and perpetrators of collective violence.

INVISIBLE TENTACLES

The guardsmen, the police, the courts, the UCEP "sharks," and the prisons are "the somber and stern face" that the Argentine state turns toward "the dispossessed and dishonored categories trapped in the hollows of the inferior regions of social and urban space" (Wacquant 2009: xviii). Shantytown dwellers and residents of squatter settlements and ill-reputed housing projects live at the margins of the social and spatial structure and survive in the cracks and crevices of a rapidly gentrifying city. For these populations, as well as for those who dare to rebel against oppressive living conditions, the Argentine state deploys open repression, imprisonment, illegal violence, and what without a hint of irony the city government's chief of staff calls "slow and silent" expulsion.

Together with its iron fist and its clandestine kicks, the state also uses softer, less visible "tentacles" to keep the urban pariahs under control. To illustrate this, let's return to a typical eviction scene. At the eviction, we find police personnel, judicial officials, and UCEP enforcers that constitute the masculine, repressive right hand of the state, as well as agents that belong to the state's feminine left hand (Bourdieu 1999), the officials from the Ministerio de Desarrollo Social, the state welfare agency. What are they doing there? To answer this, I reviewed a number of cases drawing upon informal interviews with state officials, fieldwork at the welfare agency in the city of Buenos Aires, and newspaper coverage, and in so doing I uncovered a basic logic. Welfare agents, who are usually less noticeable than repressive forces, make themselves present during most evictions in order to encourage the recently expelled to apply for a "housing subsidy" available from the state welfare agency. As mentioned above, sometimes those evicted are given some cash on the spot and asked to apply to the program immediately. The cash amount of this subsidy varies according to the number of members in the household, but it usually covers no more than six months of rent in one of the rundown hotels in the city. On occasion, the subsidy is utilized as a bribe to entice intruders to leave the illegally occupied property. When the bribe for whatever reason does not work, UCEP enforcers step in. The irony here is that like a racketeer, the state produces a danger—through eviction it creates a homeless population—and then, at a price, offers a precarious and limited shield against it (Tilly 1985). The price to be paid is the often-silent submission of the poor to the mandates of the state.[16]

In the immediate aftermath of an eviction, a new ordeal begins for the now homeless population. It is the common experience of those who for a variety of reasons end up in the welfare office and of those at the lower rungs of the social and cultural space who frequently have to interact with numerous state agencies. Like Josef K. in Kafka's *The Trial*, every time the dispossessed seeks a solution from a state agency to his or her pressing problems of housing, food, and environmental hazards (Auyero and Swistun 2009), he or she is likely to become progressively entangled in the state's web of power. This web is composed of uncomfortable waiting rooms and corridors, ever-changing paperwork, and long and unpredictable delays. During this ordeal, the physical violence of the visible fist takes a back seat, and a less evident form of domination begins to operate. The impossible requests, grueling runabouts, sudden and unexplained cancellations, and other such delay tactics are the "tentacles" that poor people can't quite see and that produce *routine* outcomes nobody explicitly intends. A subtler production of poor people's compliance occurs through the manipulation of the time of those in need, in contrast to the more visible deployment of force and control of bodies and spaces. In the vignette given earlier in this chapter, Jessica essentially describes the manufacturing of patients of the state: she and others like her just "sit and wait" and "keep coming, and wait, wait, wait." They experience endless postponements because of bureaucratic mistakes, inattentions, and random rectifications because of the perennial underfunding of the presumably benign arm of the state.

We first met Mónica at the waiting room of the welfare office with her two-year-old child in tow. She was waiting for a resolution on her housing subsidy, and this was her third time in the office. A national from Peru, Mónica is also a legal resident of Argentina. She was evicted the previous month from a squatter house and had been receiving the subsidy for a month, but, as she explains it: "One day they didn't give me any more. They told me that I had incomplete documents. They wanted a certified letter of eviction on part of the owner." This is the kind of precarious, itinerant life lived by many of the people we met at the office, and it captures in elementary and absurd detail the workings of the state's less visible exercise of power. Mónica's story continues as follows:

> MÓNICA: I lived in a *casa tomada* [squatter house]. I rented a
>   room, because they didn't want to rent to me with him [her
>   two-year-old son], they don't like to rent with babies . . . When

they evicted us I had a friend who told me that I could move to her place, share the room with her until I found something else.

INTERVIEWER: That's how you arrived here?

M: Yes, because a man during the eviction told me to come here, that here they would help me rent something . . .

I: And that's how you entered the housing program [Plan Habitacional]?

M: But they only gave it to me for the first month. Every time I came back they told me to come on another date, that the payment still wasn't resolved.

I: What explanations did they give you?

M: At the beginning they told me that the day of payment for foreigners still wasn't scheduled. But later they told me that they didn't give it to me because I lacked documentation.

I: What documentation?

M: A letter. A certificate of eviction signed by the owner of the place where they evicted me from, which I never could obtain [emphasis that Mónica signaled with her hand].

I: Because . . . ?

M: Because I never met the owner.

I: So . . . first they evicted you, they recommended that you come here, they gave you a month of subsidy, and then they didn't just stop paying you but they told you to bring a certificate of eviction after having evicted you?

M: Uh huh.

As I stated earlier, the character of the interactions between the poor and the state (and the resulting poor people's submission) described in this book is not the result of a master plan, nor can it be attributed to actors behaving in a more or less efficient manner or in typical terms of a means to an end. Just like the more visible fist, these invisible tentacles do not obey a sure-handed implementation of a foresighted plan. Instead, they constitute a "strategy (of domination) without a strategist" (Bourdieu and Wacquant 1992). Poor people's compliance therefore results from the complex interactions of the many actors involved. These interactions draw upon accumulated shared understandings, which regard both how state agencies work and the ways in which poor people have always obtained resources (i.e., after long waits). It is these understandings that crucially limit what they think, feel, and do.

In the chapters that follow I will argue, by presenting empirical evidence to that effect, that repeated trips to state offices and inter-actions with state officials and courts teach poor people that if they are to get a hold of resources crucial to their survival, they will have to *comply by waiting, usually silently*. These interactions include injunctions such as "sit down and wait"; friendly and not-so-friendly advice such as "come back in a month and we'll see"; and also human mistakes, delays caused by computer crashes, errors in understanding state language, and routine corrections of time limits produced by chronic underfunding and administrative errors. On a daily basis, this strategy of domination re-creates the asymmetry between urban denizens and state agents, and subordinates the former by routinely "inducing anxieties, uncertainties, expectations, frustrations, wounds and humiliations" (Bourdieu 2001: 110).

As Loïc Wacquant, in his insightful synthesis of materialist and symbolic approaches to penality, writes: "The police, courts, and prison are not mere technical implements whereby authorities respond to crime —as in the commonsensical view fostered by law and criminology—but a core political capacity through which the state both produces and manages inequality, identity, and marginality" (2008: 13). The iron fist of the Argentine state indeed has this dual role, as do the other forms of state power. They act to "enforce hierarchy and control contentious categories" by removing the homeless from public plazas, evicting the poor from squatted property, jailing and/or physically harassing poor youngsters living in shantytowns and other destitute neighborhoods, and besieging public projects with the national guard. They also, Wacquant notes, "communicate norms and shape collective representations and subjectivities" (2008: 13) by fueling perceptions of "young predators" who can only be controlled with *mano dura*, classifying certain poor as "undeserving" of a place to live and "deserving" of violent cleanup operations, and molding patients of the state as opposed to rightful citizens.

As I write this, hundreds of residents of the city and state of Buenos Aires are protesting in front of the federal Ministerio de Desarrollo Social in an effort to claim their right to participate in a work program recently created by the government. In drawing upon a collective action tactic that has become quite common in the last two decades in Argentina (Svampa and Pereyra 2003; Auyero 2007), they are camping in front of the main office of the Ministerio and blockading traffic in the Avenida 9 de Julio, Buenos Aires's main artery (*Clarín*, November 3, 2009; *Página12*, November 4, 2009). In no way do I suggest that the three forms of poverty regulation presented above achieve complete domination of the dispossessed. The attempt to manufacture acquiescence is always partial, always negotiated. Three decades of neoliberal economic policies continuously generate enough misery on the lower side of the social and physical space that it is hard to imagine an end to disorders generated by structural adjustment. As social insecurity multiplies, so will unrest; and so will the diverse operations of the state's exercise of power.

Patricia is very angry. She left her four children (twelve, ten, eight, and four years old) alone at home in order to come to the welfare office. She began the paperwork for the Nuestras Familias program four months ago but she has not been admitted yet. "The employees treat you badly here. When you ask them a question, they answer in a rude way. They don't care because all the people here are poor, they are all in need. Even when you cry, they don't care." She first came to the welfare office to do the paperwork for the program Ciudadanía Porteña, which she received when she was living in Villa Cartón. Today, she hopes to receive some news about the Nuestras Familias through a friend whose brother works at the welfare office. If you don't know somebody inside, she believes, your papers end up in a drawer and nobody looks at them (los cajonean, as she puts it). "If you are alone," she tells us, "you can't do anything. There're people who come early in the morning and they left in the afternoon, without any news, tired of so much waiting. Last Friday I waited for four hours, I missed the end of the year celebration at my son's school. I wanted to leave at noon but they told me to wait here because nobody knew exactly what was going on with my paperwork." As she points to the crowd sitting in the waiting room, she says: "Look at people's faces, people leave this office very, very tired."

A blazing fire that began in the early morning hours of February 8, 2007, destroyed the homes of three hundred families in Villa Cartón (Cardboard Shantytown), located beneath Highway 7 in the city of Buenos Aires. According to newspaper reports, emergency rescue vehicles assisted 177 residents of the shantytown. The following day the federal fire chief told reporters that he was investigating "arson." Weeks later, Gabriela Cerruti, then minister of human and social rights of the city government, confirmed in a press release the fire chief's suspicions, and denounced the "political intentionality of the fire." A barrage of accusations then erupted between different political factions, some within the city government and others within the federal government. Each accused the other of "manipulating the poor," or "using the poor to advance positions," and each group decried the purported connections between the arsonists and "people in power." Other officials familiar with the events of February 8 confirmed the premeditated nature of the fire. For example, the chief of police sardonically intoned, "Can you imagine, not even a drunkard was caught *desprevenido* [off guard]? So, [clearly] most people in the shantytown knew about this beforehand."[1]

The case of Cartón vividly illustrates one way in which clandestine kicks operate in the daily life of the urban poor. In this case, the kicks come not from UCEP members but from neighborhood brokers with well-oiled connections to established members of the polity. Cartón shows us precarious living conditions in their extremes, and in doing so it also exemplifies how in the aftermath of a disaster the dispossessed become ensnared in the workings of the state's invisible tentacles.

EQUINE PARADOX

When the state prosecutor Mónica Cuñarro investigated the shantytown fire in Villa Cartón, she faced, in her words, "quite a paradox."[2] Horses and carts, which are some of the "most important working tools of the local population" who scavenge the streets of Buenos Aires as a means of subsistence, were surprisingly absent when the fire engulfed the shantytown. If the fire had been an accident, would not many of the horses and carts have been caught in the inferno? Indeed, the prosecutor noted that the horses' absence was one of the many signs proving the preplanned character of the fire, along with the fact that the residents of the shantytown "avoided [other] vital losses [including] goods such as appliances, chairs, desks, etc." She concluded

that the "neighborhood leaders planned the fire, and informed most of
the local residents who, at around 5 A M, removed appliances, clothing,
and mattresses from their houses and moved the horses [to safety]" in a
nearby field, which was owned by a relative of a political activist from a
faction opposing the acting mayor. Cuñarro's report also notes that
much of the damage from the fire could have been prevented had
anyone from the shantytown called the fire department. Even though
there were cell phones available to make such a call, no one had both-
ered. Contrary to what was reported initially by the media, the report
states that "a further element of proof is that . . . luckily, there were no
fatal victims, no one was burned, no one suffocated, no one was hos-
pitalized . . . [showing] that the residents were mere spectators of the
fire. There were no victims or material losses because, since they knew
what was going to happen beforehand, they were able to protect themselves and safeguard their valuables."

    In the weeks and months following the arson and Cuñarro's report,
a torrent of public finger-pointing ensued. Opposing political factions
openly accused each other of engaging in a "dirty political campaign,"
while the minister of human and social rights accused one official
linked to the federal government of masterminding the arson. Then, in
August 2007, six months after the incident, the state prosecutor asked
a judge to indict a grassroots activist who was a member of one of the
political parties campaigning against the mayor. Although the judge
refused the prosecutor's request, citing lack of solid evidence, the report produced by Cuñarro is nonetheless revealing in that it points
unambiguously to the links between those who were directly responsible for starting the fire and the maneuverings of well-established political actors.[3] She writes: "We cannot ignore the fact that the episodes
were planned for a time that was close to the elections in the city, and
that they were planned by neighborhood leaders who wanted to use a
massive disaster in order to put pressure on local authorities to either
obtain housing or subsidies." Further, the report points to the potential connection between the events in Villa Cartón and other episodes
of collective violence in the city, such as the organized invasion of an
unfinished housing project in Bajo Flores that took place less than two

months after the episodes in Cartón (*Clarín*, April 17, 2007). Specifically, the report finds that in the months preceding the local elections there had been a dramatic increase in these episodes of seemingly
planned collective violence throughout the city, a fact corroborated by
several newspapers. What was the cause of the increase in this probably
orchestrated collective violence?

According to informal conversations and interviews with former
state officials and the prosecutor from the Villa Cartón case, party
activists, such as those who were implicated in the shantytown arson
and the invasion of the unfinished housing project in Bajo Flores,
typically hoard access to the subsidies, housing, and food packages
distributed by state agencies. They do so through their control of the
government's registries of beneficiaries, keeping track of who receives
government subsidies, housing, or food packages. These local leaders
decide who "makes it" onto the registry and who does not. In an
interview, one former local official described how the process works:
"When we were trying to register shantytown dwellers for Ciudadanía
Porteña (a welfare plan), we would open an office in each shantytown,
and in many a case nobody showed up. Only after clearing things up
with the local leaders would people begin to register. These local leaders told us: 'Just open the office, and they will come.' Obviously, they
are the ones who keep control of the final list."[4] In other words, local
leaders, not state officials, are the ones who tell the local population
when and where to register for a welfare plan, and when *not* to heed the
announcements of public officials who, as the local population sus-
pects, might use a register to collect data that will later be used to
evict them or to deprive them from other benefits. In this way, well-
connected local leaders attempt to *control the timing of the state's always precarious and always limited welfare programs*. The state prosecutor explained it this way:

> Whoever controls the (welfare) registry, controls who gets the hous-
> ing, [and] under what conditions. Whoever controls the census,
> controls the state subsidies. These state subsidies are arbitrarily dis-
> tributed, nobody checks them, they are not centralized . . . Those

who have the neighborhood registry and the subsidies obtain the control over that particular territory, they are the ones who decide who comes into the shantytown and who has to leave, who gets the bricks and other materials (for building) and who doesn't.[5]

The recently appointed mayor, who was formerly the vice mayor and had taken office after the previous mayor was impeached, announced that he would run for reelection. After his decision, one of his first projects was aimed at creating some order in what many saw as a chaotic city welfare administration. His decision to "rationalize"—or, less euphemistically, to recover control over—local welfare registries triggered a series of events leading up to the election, such as the fire in Villa Cartón and the invasion of the housing project in Bajo Flores. By generating episodes of collective violence, local leaders expressed in no uncertain terms that they were not going to give up control over state resources in their territories, just as they were not going to give up the attendant power that came with that control. In the words of the state prosecutor's report, the objective of the arson was to "completely destroy the place as a way of exerting pressure on local authorities [the mayor and the municipal officials in charge of housing policies]." What were the arsonists trying to accomplish? In her report and in a subsequent interview, the state prosecutor made it quite clear what the arsonists were up to: they were "trying to . . . acquire housing." By burning down the shantytown, they would force municipal officials to move the now homeless population to the top of the list of those waiting for public housing. They were also seeking to *speed up the passage of (waiting) time for their destitute followers*. In analytical terms they enacted clandestine kicks to avoid being ensnared in the state's concealed tentacles.

With a huge and increasing public housing deficit, where thousands of residents are awaiting for an apartment in one of the units the city administration is slowly building (CELS 2009; Defensoría de la Ciudad 2009), only a dramatic disruption of the queue can move new applicants to the top. The arson that left hundreds of families homeless is just such a disruption; and in the short term, the perpetrators seemed to have enjoyed some success in hastening government action. By late February 2007, at the beginning of a highly contested political campaign that they would eventually lose, administration officials made the Cartón population a public housing priority. A few weeks after the fire destroyed their homes, Cartón dwellers were among the future beneficiaries of a soon-to-be-built public housing complex.

"I've been living below the highway for 21 years," the shantytown dweller Lidia told a reporter from *La Nación*. "Imagine how long I've been waiting to have a roof [Mirá si habré esperado para tener un techo]. All I want is a house, that's all" (*La Nación*, February 22, 2007). Together with twelve hundred former residents of Cartón, Lidia moved into one of the fifty-seven tents that the city government put up to house those left homeless by the fire. The provisional camp was located in Parque Roca, at the crossroad of Avenida Coronel Roca and Avenida Escalada in the Villa Riachuelo neighborhood, in the southwestern limits of the city of Buenos Aires.

Close to 150 families accepted a housing subsidy from the city government and moved on their own to a new location. One official of the current administration told us that when "Cartón happened, the subsidies came out really, really fast, like a *metralleta* [machine gun]." A majority of 336 families, however, decided to move to Parque Roca. There they would await apartments in a new public housing complex that the government had announced would soon be ready.

The living conditions in the camp were dismal: scarce potable water, few portable chemical toilets and showers, and so on. Further, the combination of overcrowded tents and the lack of available public transportation—and the subsequent isolation of its inhabitants—was a recipe for disaster. This dire situation arose less than three weeks after the fire. Norma Franco, a former resident of Cartón, was living in one of the tents when in the middle of a storm a strong wind knocked down a beam, which fell on her. She was only twenty-six years old. Beto Corral, another camp resident, told the newspaper reporter Pablo Novillo the following: "The storm began around 1 AM. The tents were flying everywhere, they looked as if made of paper, and 20 or so of them fell down. I began to help people to get out. When I reached Norma's tent, she was hugging her six-month-old baby, she was very injured" (*Clarín*, February 27, 2007).

The construction of the promised housing complex dragged on. While residents waited, they were forced to endure other queues: "Lines and lines under the sun in order to eat," Estela told us, "and we felt *incomunicado*, the access was very difficult." They had fights with city authorities because, Estela pointed out, "they mistreated us. Everything we had was wet, and those who were not included in the census [the city government conducted right after the fire] could not receive a subsidy. Some took the money [from the subsidy] and left. They were afraid."

After the storm, residents were moved from the tents to a "transitory housing" complex that the government hastily built a few blocks from the tents. Living conditions were equally miserable: there was no electricity, no potable water, and a precarious sewage system. On February 16, 2009, a judge ordered the closing of the "evacuee center." Residents were dispersed to various other locations such as hotels and existing public housing in the city. We found some of them applying for housing subsidies in the welfare offices of the city government and sharing with other denizens their grueling experience of waiting, to which we now turn.

Milagros's Trial

In the back of the welfare office waiting room, twenty-seven-year-old Milagros plays with two little children, one of whom is her two-year-old son Joaquín.[6] Milagros is Peruvian, having arrived in Buenos Aires five years ago, and has been "in this thing" (i.e., navigating the paperwork at the welfare office) for a year and a half. She is a beneficiary of two programs, Nuestras Familias and Subsidio Habitacional. The Subsidio Habitacional is "late," she tells us, "because there's no payday scheduled for foreigners." She has been told that with a national ID card "everything would go faster," but without it "there's not much they can do." She has the *precaria* (literally "precarious" resident status). Four months ago, she started the paperwork to obtain a national ID card at the RENAPER, but she has to wait "for a resolution at least one more year."

She oftentimes walks to the welfare office; it's a mile and a half walk but it saves her much needed cash. Since giving birth she can't carry much weight on her, so on the days Joaquín's grandmother can't babysit, Milagros has to take the bus with him. The expensive bus fare is not the only reason why she avoids coming with him. Waiting, she says, is "boring and tiring" for her and her son. Waiting, she adds, is "costly" because of the expenses she incurs every time her son demands "something to drink or to eat" from the little stand located in the back of the welfare area. In her nickel and dime life, a thirty-cent bus ride and a dollar treat are luxuries she can't afford. Milagros's story is not anecdotal. During one of our first observations, another mother scolded her little daughter, saying, "You are making me spend a fortune. That's it. I'll buy you a chocolate milk in the afternoon"; and we witnessed dozens of similar occasions and were told comparable stories by many interviewees.

Milagros learned about the welfare benefits from a social worker at the hospital where she gave birth. When she first attempted to apply, she came to the welfare office at dawn. "At 4 AM, they were giving thirty slots, and I was number thirty-two. I thought they were going to attend [to] me, but they didn't." The next day, she came "earlier . . . at 11 PM (the night before). I waited outside all night long but there was some sort of problem and they didn't open the office that day. That was a long wait." She then waited three more months. One day, she came back at noon and was told to come earlier in the morning. She did the paperwork and received the housing subsidy for one month. Since the owner of the apartment from whom she was renting "did not have everything in order," her subsidy was abruptly terminated. She had to start the paperwork all over again in order to receive two more installments, after which she ceased to be eligible.

Milagros makes US$9 per day taking care of an elderly couple, and she can't afford to miss a day at work. When she comes to the welfare office she meets with friends, and they talk about how agents give them the "runaround." "You feel despondent here [te desanimás]," she tells us, "because [the welfare agents] tell you to come on day x. You ask for permission at work and then you find out that they have not deposited the money. I lose one day at work . . . I think the aid is a good thing but . . . well, I don't think it's fair that they make you wait so long and that sometimes they make you come here for nothing [*te hacen venir al pedo*] . . . They tell you to come on Monday, and then Wednesday, and then Friday . . . and those are working days." Milagros does not know whether or not she will receive the subsidy today. The last time she came to this office she "left with nothing." She felt "impotent" and cried a lot at home, she tells us, but *"here I didn't say anything"* (my emphasis). She desperately needs the aid the city government offers to pay the rent and to feed her son.

In Milagros's story we see patterns repeated in the waiting experiences of other welfare recipients. Contrary to initial visual impressions regarding the solitary nature of waiting, we see that waiting is in fact doubly *relational*. First, people like Milagros learn about the available welfare benefits from trusted others, such as friends and relatives, and from social workers. Second, as in Beckett's *Waiting for Godot*, clients and potential clients awaiting a decision on their cases or a payment are usually not alone in the waiting rooms. They create or mobilize a set of relations that allow them to spend long hours there. While waiting, they oftentimes meet with friends and relatives who help them tolerate *and* make sense of those "boring and tiring" hours.

Milagros's story also teaches us that waiting is a *process*, not a single event. The overwhelming majority of those we interviewed in the waiting room of the welfare office had gone through some version of what, referring again to Kafka's Josef K., we could call "the trial" of welfare. This trial resembles other long waits in public hospitals and in other state offices. As Milagros's story of endless hassle illustrates well, this process is pervaded by *uncertainty* and *arbitrariness* and results in frustration, much like Kafka's story of waiting. Moreover, it is a process that is dominated by persistent *confusion* and *misunderstanding*.

Finally, Milagros's statement regarding what she did when forced to wait—"here I didn't say anything"—and her description of her feelings at the time—"impotent"—point to the aspect of waiting that is probably the most difficult to dissect (and the reason why I believe it should be studied in the first place): most of the time the majority of the poor people we observed and talked to ultimately put up with the uncertainty, confusion, and arbitrariness of waiting. I believe that we can find the "why" of their compliance in the "how" of it. How do they spend that "dead" time? How do they make sense of, and think and feel about, the long hours of the wait?

I will begin to examine these issues where Milagros did, at the RENAPER office. After providing a description of the place where people wait many hours a day, I will document the confusion and uncertainty pervading the process of obtaining documentation. At the RENAPER, we see an elementary form of the experience of waiting, which later we will find more developed, more extensive, and more recurrent at the welfare office and in Flammable shantytown. Looking closely at the random and unexplained changes endured by those in line, and at the confusion and uncertainty dominating poor people's viewpoints on the process, I will argue that everything in their experience of waiting conspires to teach them a lesson: "Keep waiting, be patient, there's nothing you can do about the endless queues." Those in the lower regions of the social and symbolic space learn, in practice, to be patients of the state.

In order to provide the reader with a travel guide for the ethnographic descriptions ahead, I present in the following a synthesis of the three processes that take place as poor people wait and that vary by setting.

— *Veiling*: This occurs when human actions responsible for the extensive wait times of the underprivileged are masked behind the operation of nonhuman operations, such as a computer machine or a bank deposit. For example, the command to a prospective welfare client to wait three more hours for her check is given by a person (a state agent), but no individual is presented as responsible for it. In a way logically similar to "commodity fetishism" as described by Karl Marx, machines are said to "reprogram" the client by themselves, and no human can control them.
— *Confusing*: This is when those who wait are given contradictory

and puzzling messages regarding the extent and purpose of their waiting. One example is when procedures to obtain a national identification card, which only those who lack the right connections are forced to endure, are randomly changed; another is when news about the relocation of a shantytown or a new welfare program is delivered in murky bureaucratic language.

— *Delaying or rushing*: This is when waiting periods are suddenly cancelled until "further notice" or postponed "until funds are available," or when waiters are taken by surprise and abruptly awarded a service or a promise of its imminent delivery, which they thought they would have to wait much longer to receive. Beneficiaries are, in the words of many state officials we interviewed, "kicked around." One example is when shantytown dwellers are told that relocation is imminent—"they told us we should start packing this week"—and then notified that it has been suspended with no further explanation.

Together, veiling, confusing, and delaying or rushing snare poor people into uncertain and arbitrary waiting time. This blowing hot and cold, raising expectations and then mutely crushing them, inducts poor people into a process they can neither understand nor control. Over many hours, from early in the morning until late at night, we tagged along with dozens of individuals while they interacted with different state agencies or as they were waiting at home for their "Godot" (i.e., a subsidy, an ID, a relocation plan). We were there as dispossessed agents became, much like Kafka's Josef K., ensnared in the state's web of obscure and arbitrary proceedings, in effect surrendering to the time frame of the state.

THE RENAPER

The office of the RENAPER is located in an early twentieth-century stone building that looks like many public offices in the city of Buenos Aires. Legal residents of Argentina come to this office to acquire a Documento Nacional de Identidad (national ID card, hereafter DNI).

Much like a driver's license in the United States, a DNI is needed for almost every official or unofficial procedure in Argentina, including access to programs distributed by the welfare office. As Cristian, a national from Paraguay, confided to us as he was waiting in line: "Without the DNI you can't do anything. You can't get credit, you can't buy appliances . . . I need it, I can't pay cash." When Verónica obtained her DNI after coming to the office four times (they kept telling her something was missing in her application), she happily told us: "I will now be able to receive my pension!"

In order to set up an appointment to acquire a DNI, the resident needs to have a *resolución de residencia* (residence ruling) dictated by the Dirección Nacional de Migración. Many stories in national newspapers have chronicled the waiting period in that office, and in noting the day-long waiting lines officials have spoken of it as a "collapsed system."

With the "residence decision in hand," legal residents go to the RENAPER. The office opens at 6 AM, and starts giving "appointments" on a first-come, first-served basis until 10 AM. The office then closes and reopens from 6 PM to 10 PM to give a second round of appointments, again on a first-come, first-served basis. On average, appointments were given for seven months in the future, but during our four months of observation, this waiting time would extend to nine months. The day of the appointment, the resident has to present a number of documents to the RENAPER officials. If all the documents are in order, residents have to wait another four months to acquire their DNI. This admittedly cumbersome process is made even more excruciating by the fact that the "office hours," the "waiting order," and sometimes the documents solicited to acquire an appointment are often altered without notice. As a result, the size of the line can never be predicted. Sometimes we found two hundred people waiting outside the RENAPER, other times on the same day of the week and time of day we found a dozen (see fig. 2).

There are two areas for the waiting population: the sidewalk and the covered hall of the RENAPER. During the course of our fieldwork,

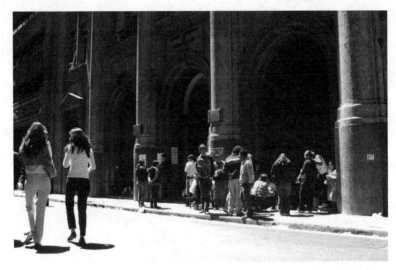

2 Waiting outside the office of the Registro Nacional de las Personas (RENAPER).
Courtesy of Agustín Burbano de Lara.

waiters were only occasionally allowed to wait inside the office. As
figure 2 shows, the sidewalk outside of the RENAPER is very narrow
(1.5 meters wide). As we will see, a long line can be formed anytime
between 6 AM and 5 PM, and when there are people in line the sidewalk is completely occupied. Passersby are forced to walk on the streets
with the obvious risk of an accident, given that in downtown Buenos
Aires there is a high volume of traffic (buses, cabs, trucks, bicycles,
mopeds, and scavengers' carts) between 8 AM and 6 PM.

Waiting on the sidewalk or in the hall is very uncomfortable. There
are no chairs, and people have to sit and sometimes sleep on the floor
using cardboard pieces they bring or find nearby. We recorded many
instances of what could readily be called the "indignities of waiting":

August 29, 2008, noon:[7] A family of four (two kids, around four and seven) are
eating "in line." They are sitting on the floor, on top of a piece of cardboard.
They are eating crackers, rice, and chicken, they also have a few bananas and
they all share a two-liter bottle of Pepsi. They place the garbage inside a
bag, on the floor, next to their food . . . Inside a hall adjacent to that of the

RENAPER, people wait in line sitting on the marble staircase of another public office. A mother is changing her baby's diapers on the stairs.

September 4, dawn: I arrive to the RENAPER at 5:25 AM. Under the gates' threshold, a huge comforter protects Jesús and his wife from the cold. They arrived at 11 PM yesterday. My steps wake up the wife and she sticks her head out. She smiles . . . she has a sleepy face. Jesús's face is not covered by the comforter and it seems to me that he has not slept during the night. "The things we have to do . . . no?" he tells me. There's another couple three meters from them; they have arrived at 3 AM. At 5:40 AM there are sixty-five people in the line, among them four small children . . . At 7 PM, the temperature is 2 degrees Celsius . . . it is very difficult to take fieldnotes, my hands are freezing.

Not infrequently, these indignities extend to the treatment that waiters receive from RENAPER personnel, who "tell us to fuck off." As Carmen, a thirty-five-year-old woman from neighboring Paraguay, told us: "Right in front of my face the guards closed the doors. Together with a bunch of mothers, we begged them to let us in, because we have the babies. And they didn't let us in. They told us that if we want to be attended to, we need to wake up earlier. I have a nine-month-old baby, and I have to travel an hour and a half to get here. The guard didn't believe me."

Waiters are not alone during the long hours of wait outside the office. Street sellers cater to this waiting population in two ways. They sell food and drinks (soda, coffee, sandwiches, and regional food like *chipas*) along with the ID pictures that waiters will use in their applications for the DNI. Pictures are not really needed because they can be taken inside the RENAPER, and a small sign outside the building indicates so. Yet nobody pays much attention to it; and given that procedures frequently change so abruptly it is quite understandable that the sign is routinely ignored. Street sellers take advantage of the almost total absence of information that is a hallmark of this waiting area to convince applicants of the need of a "nice ID picture," and they usually charge three or four times what applicants would pay inside. As one street seller confided to us after he had seen us many times in line, and after we had told him the purpose of our visits: "Given that you've been honest with me, I'll be honest with you: No, you don't need a picture ID to get an appointment, but I have to make a living and this is much better than working at a car wash. There they pay you fifty pesos for twelve hours of work, and here I work seven hours and I make eighty pesos. I get paid for every person I bring into the store [to take their picture]." Occasionally, waiters vent their frustration with the long and unpredictable line by accusing these street sellers of cheating them, even though they rarely challenge state officials. In fact, only twice did we witness loud complaints against RE-NAPER bureaucrats.

People in line are overwhelmingly from lower-income sectors of the city of Buenos Aires and from greater Buenos Aires. They spend their waiting time, which can sometimes take up to eight hours, eating, drinking, chatting, sitting on the sidewalks, standing up with their bodies leaning on the stone walls, or sleeping. The brief descriptions below point to one defining feature of the wait outside of the RENAPER: to wait, to "make it" until one is attended to, is to *endure, to not give up.*

August 29, morning: People sit on the floor, staring nowhere in particular. A couple of them have fallen asleep. Others are standing up, leaning on the wall. They don't talk much to each other. Every now and then they review the documents they have ready to hand in when their time comes, as if to make sure they have not forgotten anything—after so many hours in the line, the idea of not having all the required papers seems to assault their minds.

September 15, 2 PM: It's Monday, there's more people in line, more vendors, more garbage on the sidewalk, more traffic on the street than usual. People look tired, there are a lot of people fast asleep, many of them are sitting on the floor. There are more kids, more babies, more food around than usual. I count 162 people in line. Today, doors were not opened at noon, as done last Thursday. Guards did not tell people that this was going to be the case. They inform them that doors will open at 6 PM (but the doors opened at 4:10 PM).

September 15, 4 PM: Today people look really uncomfortable in line. I counted five asleep, and twenty or so are struggling to keep awake. According to one of the vendors, fifteen people left the line after they were not give appointments at 8 AM. They abandoned, they quit. They couldn't take it.

Third week of October, afternoon: At least a hundred people in line. Eyes half-opened, bodies as if spilled onto the walk, lethargic yawns, necks moving in slow motion . . . looking nowhere in particular.

"Punitive sanctioning through the imposition of waiting," writes Barry Schwartz "is met in its most extreme forms when a person is not only kept waiting but is also kept ignorant as to how long he must wait" (1975: 38). Legal residents of Argentina who wait in line outside the offices of the RENAPER to obtain their DNI not only have to wait long hours to start their *trámite* (paperwork), but also—and most importantly for my argument in this book—are kept in the dark regarding the length of their wait and the exact paperwork needed for a successful acquisition of an ID. The "not quite knowing" is coupled with a radical arbitrariness regarding ever-changing procedures and the absolute lack of a predictable "waiting period." One brief fieldnote excerpt recorded as we were beginning our fieldwork in August 2008 encapsulates the unpredictability of the line at RENAPER: "Two hundred people are waiting outside the RENAPER. They have been waiting since roughly 8 AM. At 2 PM, the guards inform them that they are going to open the office doors at 6 PM. At 4:30 PM, with no particular announcement, the doors are opened and all of those who have been waiting are attended to. I ask the guards what's going on and they tell me that 'today is an exception because it's very cold outside.'" In four months of observation, we learned that what at the time we thought was a kind consideration on the part of state officials was in fact a defining feature of the process of obtaining a DNI. Contrary to what the guards told us, the RENAPER is always "exceptional": that is, according to the *Oxford English Dictionary*, "out of the ordinary course, unusual, special." During our many days and nights outside the offices of the RENAPER, we only ever observed what we oxymoronically called *regular exceptions.* We were never able to predict what was going to happen during the waiting time, or if there was even going to be a waiting time, even when we conducted observations at similar times and days of the week. The reason for this is simple: procedures for requesting an appointment kept changing, as did the actual organization of the line. The people outside of the RENAPER did not know what to look forward to because the elementary answers to the basic questions of the trámite (At what time does the office open? How long shall I expect to wait in line to be attended to? What other documents do I need?) change frequently without much notice. The average waiting time outside the office varies dramatically from week to week. Long waits are suddenly and unexpectedly interrupted by officials rushing people into the office, taking even the most prepared of observers by surprise.

The generalized feeling of "not knowing what to expect" that we detected throughout our fieldwork among legal residents who desperately need their DNI should thus be understood as a result of the only predictable element in the line: the total absence of any routine. The RENAPER shows how arbitrariness feeds the prevailing uncertainty among those individuals who, lacking connections, await services from state bureaucracies. As officials keep changing the modalities of the waiting time, powerless patients of the state are treated, much like Josef K., with "strange carelessness or indifference" (Kafka 1998: 39), and are kept ignorant as to when and how their wait will come to an end. If forcing others to wait is an integral part of the implementation of power (Bourdieu 1999), then the unpredictable dynamics of the waiting line outside the RENAPER reveal a particularly insidious, though seemingly banal, form of this exercise.

NOT KNOWING

Serenita came to Argentina eleven years ago from Paraguay. On September 11, 2008, she woke up at 5 AM and, after a ninety-minute bus ride, arrived at the RENAPER at 7 AM. She is the first person in line when we talk to her at 2 PM. She has been outside the RENAPER for seven hours now and she is quite annoyed. Early in the morning she entered the building, and when it was her turn—her "moment," as she puts it—the employee at the counter told her that they were not giving any more appointments and that she had to come back in the afternoon. Serenita embodies the indignities of waiting: it had been raining on and off and her hair, clothes, and shoes are all wet. When we talk to her, she tells us that, despite her visible distress, she does not want to leave so as not to lose her turn. The following exchange reiterates some of the elements already described about the waiting outside of the RENAPER. It also points to what is, for us, one of its defining features: the lack of accurate information that translates to a generalized uncertainty pervading the waiting experience.

> SERENITA: They should give out numbers so that one can go back home, have a tea or a coffee, have lunch, go back to work or, at least, change clothes . . .
>
> INTERVIEWER: Did they give you good information? How did you find out about the time when they are open?
>
> S: No. *I don't know anything.* The vendors tell you one thing. *We, the people, don't know how it is.* And the guards are only useful to *mandarte a cagar* [tell you to fuck off] [my emphasis].

Right then, a guard comes out of the RENAPER and orders us to straighten the line. We move. After no more than thirty seconds the guard goes back in, and we go back to our previous positions . . . "This is the ugliest waiting," Serenita tells us.

Typically, people in line do not know the exact time when the office is going to open and are never sure about the exact documents they need to bring in order to successfully apply for a DNI. If, as Sudhir Venkatesh (2002) argues, the way in which informants see and talk about the ethnographer can tell us something about the universe under investigation, then one pretty reliable indicator of the lack of objective information is that many times the waiters, who would see us shuttling back and forth in the line, would place us in the position of trusted informant. People in line recurrently asked us about the required documents and the times in which the office will open. The following dialogue with Rumilda, a national from Bolivia, illustrates this central aspect:

> RUMILDA: Do I need to make photocopies? Maybe they ask for them and, if I don't have any, they won't give me the appointment and then I'll have to come back [this is the third time she is here]. Can you keep my place in the line while I go and make copies?
>
> INTERVIEWER: Sure. But you don't need the copies.
>
> R: You never know. Did you already get an appointment? Are you sure they are not asking for copies?

In this context of the widespread absence of accurate knowledge, street sellers play the similar role of self-interested informants:

> *August 27*: The line is eighty-six people long. The first ones have arrived at 7:30 AM but by 9 AM they have not been attended to, so they decided to stay until 6 PM when the doors will be reopened again to give out appointments. . . . Throughout the course of the observation (from 11:35 AM to 2:45 PM) no guard or state official comes out to inform them or put some order in the waiting line. Street vendors are in charge of the organization of those in line—they tell the newcomers where to wait and, in the process, they try to obtain a client (by persuading them of the need to have an ID picture ready) . . . Information is scarce here. Agapito, a man from Bolivia who knows that street vendors are lying about the need of pictures, is not sure about the necessary paperwork for the appointment. "Do you need a birth certificate?" he asks, "A proof of residence? You never know," he tells me.

ARBITRARINESS

At the RENAPER there is a reason for the not-knowing (How long we will have to wait? What documents do we need?), or in other words, the generalized uncertainty of the waiting experience. Waiters do not know what to expect because the RENAPER procedures to obtain a DNI keep changing, usually in sudden, unexpected, ways. *Subjective uncertainty finds its roots in objective unpredictability.*

Waiters believe the RENAPER "is so bureaucratic" and they understand bureaucracy as an organization that is "filled with obstacles." Contrary to what the waiters think, the RENAPER is in fact the opposite of the Weberian bureaucracy—that "stable, strict, intensive, and calculable administration . . . capable of attaining the highest degree of efficiency" (1978: 223). Similar to the welfare office examined in the next chapter, "precision, stability, stringency of its discipline, and reliability" (223) are nowhere to be found in the RENAPER.

In what follows I present in chronological order excerpts from our observations and dialogues with the waiters. I then offer a brief depiction of the many procedural changes we witnessed in order to capture the absolute lack of predictability that governs the waiting time at the RENAPER, and that in turn explains waiters' generalized uncertainty. At the risk of reiterating what has been stated above, I choose to reproduce the excerpts because I think ethnographic description should privilege "showing" more than "telling."

> *September 11*: A woman from Paraguay obtains her appointment even when she doesn't have the birth certificate with the *apostille* [official seal of approval]. Today, I meet Vicky. She is here for a second time because the first time she came they denied her an appointment because her birth certificate was missing the apostille.

During the first forty-five days of observations, the number of people in line before 6 AM and between noon and 4 PM has been pretty consistent: less than 100 in the first case, and between 150 and 250 in the second. On September 12, we recorded this fieldnote:

> The outside of the RENAPER looks pretty empty when I arrive at 2 PM, there are only thirty-three people waiting. It has not been like this before. The first one in line arrived at noon. Apparently, there have been changes in the office. There's now no waiting area around the information counter, and another counter has been added to give out appointments. The doors opened from 12:30 PM to 1:30 PM today and the line got much smaller.

A few days later, we registered the following:

> At 3:47 PM, there are seventy-four people in line. Guards are telling the people that the doors will be open at 6 PM. I don't understand why they are saying this if the doors sometimes (like they did today) open at 4 PM. I asked the guard what's going on and he tells me that "many things changed since the new director took over earlier this week."
>
> *September 24*: This is Nilda's fourth time here. It took her two one-hour long bus trips and a long walk to get here from her home in the poor barrio of San Francisco Solano. She says, "On the third time, they gave me the wrong office hours because they have changed. We used to be able to wait inside, in the waiting room, but now we have to stay outside as if we were dogs . . . My legs are hurting . . . If you don't come here to ask, you won't find out any-thing. You have to come and ask. . . ."

Similarly, Juan, a sixty-five-year-old man from Paraguay who could not make it the day of his appointment because he was sick, tells us: "They told me I had to wait in line again. . . . Last time I came here, the office was open from 3 PM to 5 PM. But now they've changed."

> *September 26*: Dialogue with Lucy (forty years old, from La Paz, Bolivia):
>
> LUCY: See . . . they gave me the appointment for June 29 of next year.
> INTERVIEWER: Is this the first time you came for an appointment?
> L: Yes, but I came today at 7:40 AM and the woman in the office told me that they have already given three hundred appointments and that I should come back at 6 PM.
> I: [not understanding why they have not told her to come back at noon, given the recent changes]: And why did you come back earlier? [It's 4:45 PM].
> L: Because I thought that if they didn't attend to me this morning, even if I came very early, I'd rather come before. I came back and asked the agent at what time it was good to come back.
> I: And what did the agent tell you?
> L: She told me to come back at noon because, *sometimes, but only some-times*, they open the office at 12 PM [my emphasis].

It was at that point in our fieldwork that, given the changes introduced in the organization of the line by the new director of the RE- NAPER, we thought that our empirical object had disappeared. The average waiting time had been reduced to less than two hours, while during our first month of multiple conversations and observations the average time was around six hours. Suddenly, there were never more than forty people waiting in line outside the offices. Two weeks later, on October 7, we recorded the following:

> Now I really don't know what to expect during fieldwork. The RENAPER changed its procedures to ask for an appointment again! I arrived at 9:30 AM and there are fifty-six people in the line . . . Everyone I ask tells me that they have to wait until 6 PM: "They told us that they will reopen at 6 PM." I speak with Andrea and José. They don't know how long they will have to wait. They don't know at what time the office opens. They think that at some point in time, the line will start moving and they will be attended to.

A few days later, one of the RENAPER guards tells us: "The new director does not like to see people waiting outside . . . Sometimes people are attended to sooner, other times later; it all depends on the number of people waiting." Against the new director's preferences, that same day we counted ninety-six people waiting outside the office at 3:30 PM. Doors were not opened to the public at noon as they had been the week before. Two additional fieldwork excerpts and an informal conversation with a few waiters plainly show the combination of uncertainty and arbitrariness characterizing the waiting line. Changes were so hasty that even we attentive observers sometimes missed the action.

> *October 21*: Heavy rain. People are allowed inside the building earlier than last week. "Why?" I asked the guard. "Is it because of the rain?" "No," he replied, "the director wanted to let them in before. When he wants them to come in, they come in."

> *October 26*: I come back to the RENAPER after the morning observation expecting a big line outside. It's 2:50 PM. And *it's empty*! There's nobody

outside. No people, no vendors, nobody! A cop tells me that: "People from the office came out and said that they'd close for the day."

October 13 [dialogue in waiting line]:

ZULLY: If the line is disorganized, one doesn't know where to stand. . . . Nine months ago, they were opening the doors from 1 PM to 2 PM. They will allow us to enter soon . . .

JUAN: They will open at 3 PM . . .

MARÍA: In the afternoons, they open from 5 PM to 8 PM. . . .

INTERVIEWER: Is this your first time here?

Z: No, I've been here before. I had an appointment for September 26, but I had a cold and couldn't make it. . . .

I: And now, are you going to lose your appointment?

Z: I don't know. I came to find that out.

M: I cannot tell the number of times I've been here. I came in March because they told me the DNI was going to be ready then. They then told me to come back in June. Then in July . . . [minutes later, Zully comes out of the office, visibly annoyed]

Z: I have to make another appointment! And I have to bring all the papers again . . . Why?! If I already gave them all the documentation the first time around!

The Kafkaesque randomness of this process is, ultimately, best illustrated by the speed with which one of my colleagues obtained an appointment. The notes taken on the day that one of the research assistants working for this project (a national from Ecuador) obtained an appointment after no more than twenty minutes of waiting are reproduced below. The fieldnote was recorded the very day after we saw Jesús and his wife, during the bitterly cold early morning hours, sleeping outside the RENAPER. They had been waiting since the night before.

I arrive at the RENAPER at 4:30 PM. Everything looks normal, except for the cold. I'm number eighty-six in line, and three babies are in line. Twenty people are waiting inside the building, the rest were allowed to wait in the entry hall, forming a line in horseshoe form . . . I'm not in the mood for talking to people today. I try to engage with a couple of people with no success . . . I decide to go back home and look for my documents. I'll take advantage of my fieldwork time to make an appointment for myself. After all, I also need the DNI. I leave the RENAPER at 5 PM with the idea of coming back and waiting in line at least until 9 PM. I return at 6:30 PM with my documents in my bag. Three people are waiting in line outside. Inside, the building is empty. Cleaning personnel are mopping the floor and rearranging chairs. . . . Those waiting outside tell me they have just arrived. It is very cold so I tell them that we should go inside. They do not trust me, they look nervous as if they are afraid of making a mistake. I convince them when I tell them that in the morning people are allowed to go inside. Once inside I head to the counter where appointments are given. The waiting area has one hundred chairs; there are no more than five people waiting. The guard stops me and tells me to wait outside. I tell him that it's blistering cold outside. He tells me that he agrees with me but that the woman who sets up the appointments likes people to wait outside. We leave, and the three people who came in with me are not happy with me! A few minutes later (6:40 PM) another woman allows us inside. One of the group who came in with me does not have her birth certificate with the proper apostille. She gets very nervous and begs for an appointment, her hands as if praying. The official tells her that it doesn't matter now but she needs to have the apostille when she comes back to start the trámite. She thanks the official. After a five-minute wait, I receive my appointment for May 18, 2009. I can't believe it. I'm in shock. It's now 6:50 PM and I have my appointment. It took a total of roughly twenty minutes to get it, but after the long lines I have been observing, day and night, it certainly feels like less than five minutes. How paradoxical this is . . . "Every Friday is like this . . . we want to leave before 10 PM," the people at the counter tell me. Who would have thought that a state dependency was going to be open on a Friday at 10 PM?

Recording the Arbitrary

August 19: Women with children are served first. A few weeks later, this preferential treatment ceases.

September 5: Agustín obtains his appointment in twenty minutes. A woman obtains hers even though her birth certificate lacks the apostille.

September 11: Those in line are not allowed to wait in the hall (it's raining today).

September 18: There's a new director at RENAPER. New office hours, no waiting room for those requesting information. Office doors open in the morning, at noon, and in the afternoon. Rumilda is denied an appointment because her birth certificate lacks the apostille.

October 22: People are allowed in the office in groups of twenty, not one by one as it was the case a week ago.

October 24: There's no more waiting outside the RENAPER. People wait inside the building in a big waiting room.

October 26: People wait outside the building, but are allowed to enter on a regular basis. Office remains open during the entire day.

November 7: People make a line outside the building. They are told that it is forbidden to wait in line outside and that they should come back at 6 PM. Officials try, unsuccessfully, to dissolve the line.

November 9: Officials now let people form a line outside—and they also allow a line in the exterior hall.

November 14: Marina gets an appointment without the apostille in her birth certificate.

November 17: The line outside (in organization of space *and* time) looks like the one observed two months ago—before change of director.

DURKHEIM IN LINE

In the context of great uncertainty and arbitrariness, people outside the RENAPER do what they know best: they form a line. Even against the commands of the state officials who "don't want to see a people waiting in the street," they stick to a script they have learned in their

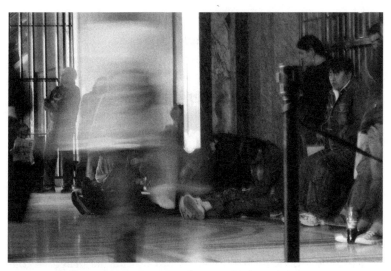

3 Line outside the RENAPER. Courtesy of Agustín Burbano de Lara.

many other encounters with state agencies such as public hospitals, the migration office, and the welfare ministry. The line as a Goffmanian interactional order also works as a veritable Durkheimian social fact. It constrains and coordinates social interaction. The fieldnote excerpt and dialogue below show us that the line is a *script that sticks*. Figure 3, taken inside the hall of the RENAPER, shows a graphic representation of that sticking script. Waiters, their bodies sitting on the floor, fixed in the line, seem to be suspended in time; while others, as if living and moving in another temporal order, pass by.

October 7, 11 AM: In the entrance hall, a small crowd is formed. After a two-hour wait outside, agents have let the people inside to tell them that the office will reopen at 6 PM. A new official—I have never seen him before—is telling them that office hours are from 6 PM to 9 PM. People leave the building and slowly begin to form a line outside. The official and the guards tell them not to form a line but rather leave and come back later. People refuse to heed their request and keep forming a line. It is as if they think, "If I want the DNI, I have to wait." A small line is now formed outside.

October 14 [dialogue in waiting line]:

MARÍA: [she did not make the cut in the morning line]: This man came out
   with two other ladies and told us that there were no more appointments
   for the morning. He told us to go away, to not wait here, he said that we
   won't get anything by waiting and that was better to return at night
   when the office is empty.

INTERVIEWER: And why did you decide to stay around?

M: Because this is not the first time that I came here. I've been in this office
   before. And see this line now? [It's 3:30 PM and there are ninety people
   in the line.] It's going to be full by late afternoon. If I stay, I win. If not, I'll
   lose two working days.

The excerpts above do not intend to account for the entire process
of acquiring a DNI. Rather, they serve to provide an analytic reconstruction of the two interrelated dimensions of the waiting process—
uncertainty and arbitrariness—that are particularly visible in the line
outside the RENAPER. State officials delay and defer, but also rush—
and take powerless state patients by surprise. In other words, they
exercise their power. The very (dis)organization of the line demonstrates the particularly denigrating or humiliating character of this
exercise. Or, to paraphrase the usher's assertion when Josef K. visits the
court office: "They show no consideration of any kind, just look at this
waiting room" (Kafka 1999: 68).

"Resignation," Pierre Bourdieu writes in *Pascalian Meditations*, "is
indeed the commonest effect of that form of 'learning by doing' which
is the teaching performed by the order of things itself" (1999: 233). In
the case of the RENAPER, this "order" is particularly chaotic. One
should thus not be surprised if those who hope to obtain a DNI form a
line and resign themselves to wait until someone at some point decides
it is time for them to enter the office. Like the welfare clients analyzed
in the next chapter, applicants at the RENAPER "just sit and wait."
Similar to the hospital for tuberculosis patients examined by Julius
Roth (1963), the waiting time is dominated by the lack of information.
Yet, different from that particular universe, here the uncertainty does

not lead to a frantic activity but to stasis, to acquiescence, or in other words to powerlessness.

It is indeed a narrative irony that this chapter relied on the stories of Milagros and Serenita, names whose literal translation mean "miracles" and "little serene," to illustrate patient waiting. Eventually, people like them do obtain their ID cards and make their way to the welfare office to ask for "help" in making ends meet. In the next chapter, we follow them there as they move through another excruciating process.

FOUR | The Welfare Office

According to official documents of the city government of Buenos Aires (Ciudad Autónoma de Buenos Aires 2008), there are twelve different programs administered at the central welfare office. However, most of the people we observed and interviewed there were waiting for a decision or a payment on one of the following three cash transfer programs: the Nuestras Familias, the Ticket Social, and the housing subsidy. The office serves Argentine nationals and documented foreigners, who are most often recent migrants from Bolivia, Paraguay, and Peru. There are no citizenship restrictions to access any of these plans, provided recipients can show proof of residence in the city of Buenos Aires.

The welfare waiting room is much like the daily life of many poor neighborhoods in the city; that is, it is a universe where Argentines and migrants from neighboring countries come together in what Erving Goffman (1961) would call a "focused gathering" (a set of individuals involved in a common flow of action, and who relate to each other in terms of that flow). Above all, however, the waiting room is a world of women and children who are seeking urgent help, and who live in "a state of emergency" (Ehrenreich 2001). Many of the women are raising their children alone or with the help of family members other than the children's fathers. In fact, the father's desertion was cited by many as the main reason why they "ended up" asking for one or more welfare benefits, while another frequently cited reason was personal illness or that of partners. Predictably, those seeking a housing subsidy come to the welfare office after an eviction. As I have already described, many of these individuals were informed by state personnel about the housing subsidy during their evictions, either from illegally occupied houses or from rental properties they couldn't afford.

Similar to the welfare rooms examined by Sharon Hays in *Flat Broke with Children*, the central office of Buenos Aires is characterized by the "ubiquity of children." Also much like Hays describes, the landscape is dominated by "the cries of hungry or frustrated or sad or disgruntled children, the laughter and chatter of playing children, the 'inconvenience' of children whom you trip over, children who are seeking amusement, and children who demand a space in your lap" (2003: 85). Children run or crawl around on the dirty floor, and babies are fed and changed in public because there are no private places for those activities (see figs. 4 and 5). One of our early fieldnotes captures the human landscape of the waiting room, as follows:

The majority of people come with someone, some even come with the entire family, like the family of five that was sitting in the back of the room. Father, mother, and older daughter (about seven years old) drank mate with cookies. The youngest of all the kids, a baby girl of two years, sat and stood up constantly, but her mother didn't let her go much. The middle son played in the corner in the back, throwing a small circle of cardboard. Each time the disk crashed against a surface the kid shouted "goal!" as if that were always the first, although he never played with a fixed goal . . . The kids shout, walk fast, run, crawl, roll around in the trash on the ground: they play. A boy of about nine years who has come with his father jumps around giving imaginary flying kicks and punches, with a "pyew" each time that he reaches his imaginary enemies with his force. The little girl to my side, when she isn't stopped, handles the trash on the ground and puts it curiously in her mouth . . . A little boy of about five years was happily playing on the exterior patio with other girls a little older than him—girls with uniforms who came directly from school—until his father brought him inside. The boy broke out in tears when his father was called to the counter. Another boy laughed out loud while his father was carrying him on his shoulders, playing with him.

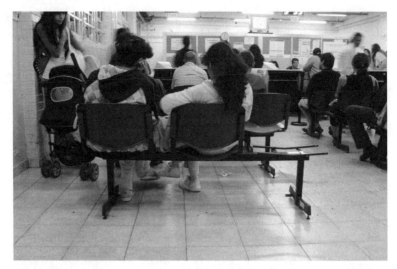

4 Waiting at the welfare room. Courtesy of Agustín Burbano de Lara.

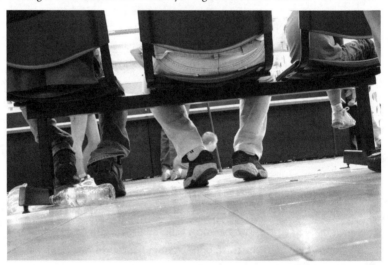

5 A baby crawling around the trash at the welfare room. Courtesy of Nadia Finck.

Megan Comfort's insightful ethnographic account of the "agonizingly long and uncertain" (2008: 50) waiting undergone in the Tube at San Quentin State Prison by inmates' wives, fiancés, girlfriends, mothers, and relatives can be used almost word by word to describe the general disposition of the bodies inside the waiting room of the welfare agency:

> Seated or standing, adults . . . pace, fidget, and rock, while their children squirm, holler, whine, and cry. Pregnant women perch awkwardly on the narrow benches, supporting their bellies with their hands because they cannot recline far enough to relieve their backs of the weight of their wombs . . . Mothers of infants clumsily assemble feeding bottles and apply fresh diapers in the absence of clean water, sanitary surfaces, or changing tables . . . [The room's] acoustics amplify and echo every outburst, squeal, tantrum, and reprimand, and visitors brace themselves against this cacophony while shivering with cold, slumping with fatigue. (45)

Comfort's description also directs our attention to the general conditions in which the waiting takes place. The waiting room at the welfare office is approximately nine meters wide and not more than twenty meters long and has only forty-eight plastic seats, counting the four or five that are normally broken, to serve a waiting population that far exceeds that number. As a result, on numerous occasions, and especially in the morning hours, the hundreds of current and potential clients passing daily through the office have to wait for hours standing, leaning against the walls, or sitting on the floor. The high windows prevent much natural light from entering the room, and therefore most of the light is provided by white fluorescent tubes. The room lacks a good ventilation system, a working heating system, and an adequate air-cooling system (out of the six existing ceiling fans, two are working). It is extremely cold in the morning hours during the winter months and unbearably hot by noon during the summer months. It is, in the words of many state officials we talked to, "an ugly place."

By the time the office closes its doors (usually around 4 PM), food remains, bottles, used napkins, spilled sodas, and even items such as used Q-tips pile up on the floors of the waiting room. Every now and then we also found vomit and dirty disposable diapers, but no cleaning personnel ever showed up during the hours we were there. After a few hours of operation, the bathrooms are also dirty, and we never found soap or toilet paper in them.

> *September 14, 2009:* There is grime on the ground from shoes. A banana peel rots at the foot of a bench, almost dressed by the remainders of mayonnaise that still remain halfway between the container and the floor. Above the place where a boy had vomited there is a ball of toilet paper piled up. Straws, candy wrappers, cartons of hot dogs with french fries, bags of french fries. The trash is concentrated in the back part of the room. In the aisles only papers are found. There are remainders of food, drinks, and wrappers at the foot of the rear benches and in the background.

> *September 16, 2009:* There is more trash on the ground at the foot of the waiting benches than in the back of the room. I find in between the posts a bottle of flavored water, a segment of mandarin, candy wrappers, round candies, mate herb. In the back aside from trash and remnants of food there is soil and the floor is dirty.

THE TEMPORAL SITE:
SOCIABILITY AMID UNCERTAINTY

Donald Roy in his now-classic piece "Banana Time" (1959) describes a group of workers who develop a series of games to deal with the "formidable beast of monotony" prevalent in their factory. Much like Roy and his coworkers, welfare clients confront a similar "beast." In almost every single one of our interviews and in innumerable informal conversations, both those held with us and those overheard, current and prospective clients refer to the tedious waiting time in terms of frustration. The following brief fieldnote excerpts summarize this shared nuisance:

October 1, 2008: A mother yells to her four-year-old who is running around: "Diana, please, stop, we have to wait." Her number is called. She comes back, and in a loud voice she tells no one in particular: "Oh, no, it can't be, it can't be . . . What are we going to do for so many hours here?!"

October 30, 2009: An eighteen-year-old (crying) tells her mother: "I hate this place . . . I'm tired of coming here, I hate the way they treat us, the things we have to do . . ."

Many current or prospective clients come to the welfare office with their children. They also come together with their neighbors or develop informal interactions in the waiting room. Clients bring and share food during breakfast and lunch time, and we frequently observed women having their meals together and sharing the care of the little ones. In a space dominated by countless urgencies regarding access to food and housing and by confusion and uncertainty about the actual workings of the welfare programs, informal interactions transmit information about existing soup kitchens, the availability and prices of housing in the city, required paperwork for a specific welfare plan, the difficulties implied in obtaining this or that document, and issues with other welfare programs distributed by the city or federal governments (i.e., which one has been, usually abruptly, canceled; which one is now accepting applicants, etc.). Although these interactions do not take the *regular form* described by Roy (I did not identify anything akin to a "banana time," a "peach time," or a "coke time"), they serve clients as a means to avoid both tedium and its "twin brother" fatigue, as Roy puts it. These interactions also informally diffuse information about formal state requirements.

While they wait, welfare clients keep themselves busy. They play with their children, they feed the little ones and change their diapers, they walk around, they leave the building for a smoke break, they buy snacks from the stand and negotiate with their children about prices and portions, they play games on their cellular phones and occasionally read the newspaper, usually the free newspapers available throughout the city in subways and kiosks. In other words, their waiting is active and relational.

Together with the informal interactions that characterize this space, a first-time visitor can easily sense the disorganization of the waiting room and the sudden changes that await those who venture there. "Let's do this," screams a welfare agent from behind the counter: "Two lines!" "Everybody against the wall," another one commands. Our fieldnotes are filled with expressions like the following, again coming from behind the counter: "Guys . . . all of those with numbers . . . please have a seat" (at the time we record this, there are no seats available). "We'll call you, but take a seat." "Please be quiet!! All those waiting for the Nuestras Familias, here . . ." "Everybody against the wall, please!" "I don't know [when you are going to be paid]. Come back in four, five, six days to know when it's your turn."

October 1, 2008: A woman comes out from behind the counter; screaming in a teacher-like voice, she says: "Let's get some order. Those who are for the Nuestras Familias, here. The rest, against the wall. They will call you by name." As a result a long line is formed in the middle of the room. Thirty minutes later, the line is dissolved. Everything is chaotic today.

The waiting room is disorganized and puzzling not only for first-time visitors but also for recurrent ones.

September 11, 2008: Two ticket counters are working today. One is on number 52, the other one signals number 47. A man from the counter is calling number 92. There's a waiting line in front of the door (and the security guards) that separates the waiting room from the offices. Plus, there's another line at the very entrance of the building. There are five different but unmarked "waiting zones" within the same room.

September 25, 2009: The noise in the room has increased. There are a few more people, a few standing, but the edge of the counter is almost clear. The family that is seated to my right watched that the turn sign is on number 58. They have number 60 and carry a filled-out paper in hand that has the title

"Reference." The woman to my left also has the same paper in hand, but her turn reads "143." She carries a one-month-old baby in her arms. The baby wakes up and begins to cry; she starts to breastfeed him. About twenty minutes later, when the baby goes back to sleep and she sees that the family that was to my right and had the same paper returns to sit by my side, she asks me, "Look, mine says 143 but the sign only has 2 numbers there." The woman to my right who has just returned says to her very certainly, "yes, yes, go, go, only the last two numbers matter, that is all that matters." "They didn't show you?" I asked. "No, I didn't know!"

October 1, 2009: A man looks at the turn sign—his turn had passed, he had 558 and the sign showed 4 63 (exactly like that, including the space), the man didn't know that they operate with only the last 2 numbers. To assure myself I ask the woman to my right and she confirms, "Yes, this already passed, it's only the last 2 numbers."

Technical malfunctions are coupled with human mistakes. We registered several instances in which beneficiaries were given appointments for days on which the office is closed. Here are two examples affecting the same person.

October 2, 2008: A woman asks me if I think Monday will be a holiday. They told her to come back on Monday (October 12 is a holiday in Argentina). I tell her that if they instructed her to come back on Monday it is because it will not be a holiday. I assume they don't give appointments for impossible days. The woman corrects me and tells me that the last time they gave her a Sunday appointment. As I later find out, she was right. They have given her an appointment for a wrong day—Monday is a holiday.

The following dialogue further illustrates the hassles and mistakes that are a constant presence in the interactions between the poor and the state, and it foreshadows some of the themes of the following pages. Ana arrived at the office at 8:30 AM on November 9, 2009. It's noon when we interview her:

INTERVIEWER: Do you know if they are going to assist you today or do you still have to wait more?

ANA: No. They gave me an appointment for December 12 [neither Ana nor the interviewer realized at the time that December 12 is a Saturday and the office is closed].

I: Appointment for what?

A: To have an interview with the social worker.

I: Are you going to begin the procedure soon?

A: No, I already received the six housing payments. But I want to ask for a renewal.

I: When did you receive the last payment?

A: This November. They gave me the last two payments together because the previous month they didn't give it to me.

I: And what is it you need for the renewal?

A: An interview with the social worker.

I: And they just gave it to you for December?!

A: Yes, because of that I came, I want to see if my friend who had to come to talk today can ask them to assist me (her friend is seated in front).

I: And what do they expect you to do in order to pay while the renewal comes out?

A: Oh I don't know, because they made the appointment for me for halfway through December. If they approve me, then they might give me the subsidy, and if they do so, it'll be when the new year is already well started.

I: What are you going to do then in order to pay rent during all of this?

A: Oh I don't know, it needs to be seen.

The waiting room is a space of "not quite knowing" what to do, what to expect, how long to wait. The fact that we were constantly used as a source of information, much like in the waiting line at the RENAPER, is again a good indication of the reigning uncertainty.

August 19, 2009: A young man of about twenty-seven years sits to my side and (referring to one of the waiting lines) asks me, "What is that for, huh?" I respond, "To apply for and receive food subsidies, like single mothers, or housing subsidies." Then more intrigued he asks me, "But it's also for men right?" "Yes, yes, also, for everyone," I reply.

The following dialogue encapsulates many of the conversations we had with beneficiaries and potential beneficiaries and sums up the uncertainty and confusion that characterizes the interactions between the poor and the state. Claudia has been waiting for four hours when we meet her in early November 2009, but we soon found out that her waiting extends further back in time:

INTERVIEWER: What plan did you come for?
CLAUDIA: For the Nuestras Familias.
I: Is today the payment day?
C: I don't know, they still don't pay me.
I: You aren't a beneficiary of the plan yet?
C: No. But a friend who started the procedure with me, the same day, has been covered two times already. And they tell me that mine isn't there.
I: How long since you came the first time?
C: I started the paperwork on the twenty-third of July, we did it together. They told us it would take about sixty days to give us a response, and it already is more than sixty days that have passed, so . . .
I: More than one hundred days in reality . . .
C: Yes, more than three months.

Even state officials working for other welfare agencies acknowledge that both the schedule and the procedures at the Ministerio are incredibly bewildering. As Susana, a Buenos Aires Presente (BAP) social worker with years of experience, told us:

INTERVIEWER: Why is there so much confusion at the Ministerio?

SUSANA: I don't know . . .

I: The beneficiaries tell us that same thing!

S: It's that sometimes we are like the beneficiaries, we don't under-
       stand why at times it's done one way and another way another
       time. [But] people wait because perhaps . . . there is a lot of
       hopelessness in that hope, as if they think, "I don't know if they
       are going to give it to me."

Random changes in procedure, scheduling, the number and cash
amount of installments, and requirements are the rule. Arbitrary
changes can be more or less consequential, as the following progression
of three different vignettes highlights:

September 14, 2009: Today people were "organized" by the employees in a
different manner than on Thursday of last week. On this occasion the en-
tirety of waiting took place in the interior of the office; today there is a police
officer who lets people enter in groups as people who are inside come out of
the place. I'm not the only person who is surprised by the external wait in
such cold weather. The woman who gets in line behind me converses with a
neighbor. A few minutes earlier they had recognized each other from one
sidewalk to the other—"You are always in a hurry!" said one woman to the
other. Upon her return I recorded the following of her conversation.

FIRST WOMAN [outside of the line]: Is it [the line] always like this? [while
    she says this she rubs her hands together as a sign of the cold]
SECOND WOMAN [in line]: No. She [another woman behind her in the
    line] came Friday and says it wasn't like this. I believe [it's like this] when
    there are many people, that's it.

September 17, 2009: Conversation in waiting line outside the welfare office:
"They haven't opened yet." "How strange, other times that I have come at
8:30 [AM] they are already attending [to people]." "But I did see people inside
through the window, even people standing." "No, they are only mothers
with their kids in arms that they let enter so they can wait sitting." "Sir, what
do the rumors in line say, are they attending [to people]?" "No, I don't know,
nobody knows."

December 7, 2009: Blanca is a recipient of the housing subsidy. She couldn't make it to the office the day in which her payment was ready and she came to reschedule it. Even when she has no complaints about the working of the office she describes a haphazard benefit.

INTERVIEWER: Were the payments always on time until now?

BLANCA: Yes, on time . . . the attention and service are good here. What happens is that they don't pay each month, they pay every other month. But every other month they pay you on time. What happens is that there isn't a fixed day to receive [the payment] but they give you like a period during which you have to come to receive [the payment], for example they say to you, "It's going to be paid between the sixteenth and the twenty-fifth," and that means that one of those days you will collect.

I: What you collect is useful to you more as an aid, it's not that if one day the payment isn't there you run the risk of them evicting you . . .

B: No, because I already know, one already knows that it's like that, as they give to you today it could be that tomorrow they don't give to you. It's here today and isn't going to be there tomorrow. You can't depend on the government, never, they have their politics today and tomorrow they will change it.

I: You're clear then that this can't be depended on . . .

B: Yes, because it can't, you can't. *If you depend on this you're dead.* [emphasis added]

Coordinators from BAP as well as social workers admit that "discretion is the rule" (*la discrecionalidad es la regla*). Below is a sample of their opinions about the workings of the welfare agency. The reader should keep in mind that these evaluations come from state agents who interact with the welfare agency on a daily basis:

"The periods [of the programs] are stipulated but aren't carried out."

"*They go stretching out the periods and they eat up a month*, without the beneficiary realizing that they aren't being covered every month" [my emphasis].

> "[Referring to the case of Villa Cartón described above] Sometimes in emergency situations like that one the subsidy is given to those affected on the spot. And then when they go to receive the second installment they find out about the requirements. Beneficiaries then learn that they can't receive a housing subsidy if they don't have their DNI. And they lose the subsidy."

In our observations and interviews with state agents and both actual and potential beneficiaries, the discretionary power of the welfare office becomes evident. Yet in contrast to the universe described by analysts of welfare bureaucracies in the United States (Watkins-Hayes 2009; Soss 1999; Lipsky 1980), this discretion in the allocation of benefits does not seem to stem mainly from the nature of the street-level bureaucracy but rather from "above"—that is, from the world of "politics." Let's listen again to BAP coordinators and caseworkers, who describe a world in which budget considerations trump all other policy decisions. This, needless to say, is not surprising:

> "When there is more money, the periods are shorter. Sometimes there is money, and they cover the subsidy the next day. It varies a lot because of the budget."

> "They change the totals according to the budget, and the quantity of quotes changes also."

What is remarkable, however, is that the discretion also originates in the world of "politics," which is understood by state agents as a world beyond their reach—as a world of obscure deals and peculiar stakes.

> "In order to remove the homeless [from a place where there's going to be an official event], money is given without them being part of any program so that they vacate immediately."

> "Suddenly there is money for a program, suddenly there isn't. If there is a massive eviction that was decided for political reasons, money appears. And the subsidy is given to the evicted at the moment of the eviction, with no requirements in mind."

"Before the elections, they give subsidies immediately, without taking the
requirements into account."

In the minds of street-level bureaucrats, elections and evictions can
shorten poor people's waiting. And they communicate so to the
beneficiaries: "We tell the beneficiaries: 'Take advantage, apply for the
subsidy, there's an election coming soon!'" Although the available data
on the monthly distribution of benefits do not show a strong correla-
tion between city elections and the distribution of resources, what is
important here is that social workers who interact with the poor on a
daily basis believe this to be the case.[1] In the case of evictions, the
available data is even sparser, since there is no database on evictions.
Yet my interviews with state officials and our observations and interviews with beneficiaries seem to confirm the diagnosis made by BAP
agents that evictions do prompt the rapid and unregulated dispensa-
tion of state resources.

Taken together, the interviews with state agents and our observations in the field confirm the statement made by one BAP coordinator that "discretion is the rule," but they also point to a larger issue.
Chronic social problems such as homelessness, precarious housing,
and hunger are routinely treated as both social and political emergencies. Ad-hoc decisions dominate much of the allocation of resources,
and are based first and foremost on political considerations such as a
rally in which the mayor is going to be present or an eviction that
is very "visible." Emergencies are, needless to say, "unstable bases on
which to ground policy" (Lipsky and Smith 1989).

As a result of this lack of clear protocol, beneficiaries are "kicked
around . . . There is a constant fumbling of people," to use BAP workers' own terms. State agents speak of *a pateo, a peloteo,* and *a manoseo*
(kicking around like a ball) of the beneficiaries, which conveys the
image of the dispossessed as things to be manipulated more than subjects with their own volition.

The welfare agency's modus operandi is, in other words, defined by
its arbitrariness. Sometimes people have to wait long hours, sometimes
not. Sometimes they are paid, sometimes not. The rescheduling of

payments is a recurrent event. One BAP social worker, all of whose beneficiaries have been rescheduled at least twice during the past three months, puts it this way: "If it is an election year, a lot of money is spent before and after elections. Then the rescheduling appears, trying to kick as much as possible, so that people give up . . . and others can hopefully be moved to the next [budgetary] year."

We asked Ana, a beneficiary of the housing subsidy, how she managed through the month in which the subsidy did not come in time. She told us the following: "I asked the landlady to let me pay her later because they had held me up with the welfare payment. She didn't make any problem for me, she knows that I'm trustworthy, that I never have ripped her off or not come through, I always pay on time." But not everybody is as lucky as Ana. Jonathan, a twenty-year-old man who lives with his nineteen-year-old girlfriend in a hotel room, tells us that when the payment is postponed "you have to sort it out with your landlord . . . you can't always tell him, 'they delay my payment, I'll pay you the rent in two weeks.' *I have to spend my time moving* [looking for another rental]" (my emphasis). We collected many stories of evictions that were caused by the state's interruption of the housing subsidy. Estela is Ana's friend and has arrived at the waiting room at 9:30 AM:

> INTERVIEWER: It's almost noon. You have already been here for more than two hours. Do you have an appointment with the social worker?
>
> ESTELA: Yes . . . I am in an emergency situation, and if they don't give me the renewal, they leave me on the street. Notice that when I first came here I already owed three months of rent, I am still owing it, because of that they threw me out of the place.
>
> I: Were you evicted? How long ago?
>
> E: They evicted me less than a month ago. With my three little ones they threw me out.
>
> I: And what did you do?
>
> E: The first night? I went to sleep at the entrance door of the Piñero Hospital. The following night I called one of the shel-

ters and they told me that they wouldn't be able to take me in because that night there was an eviction, and I returned to sleep there at the hospital.

Social workers and coordinators from BAP acknowledge that delays in payment are one of the main causes of the inability of those with unstable jobs to secure housing for long: "People stay on the street because they got behind on the subsidy"; "People return to living on the streets because the welfare office doesn't pay them on time"; "It's an atrocity because imagine that with the difficulty there is finding a hotel, getting settled, rearming your life . . . and then after three months they stop paying you because of budget shortages."

Delays and random changes, the discretionary "kicking around" in the words of the BAP coordinator, have objective consequences. Some are more serious, as when people are evicted from their hotels because of lack of payment; and others are more minor but equally aggravating, as when people lose hours of work, have to leave their children unattended at home, or miss their lunch at the local soup kitchen because of the long hours of wait and the repeated visits they have to make to the welfare office. As Frances Piven and Richard Cloward (1971) noted when they studied welfare distribution in the United States, postponements and casual alterations wear people out and discourage them from applying for other benefits they are formally entitled to. As Cebelina, a beneficiary of the Nuestras Familias told us, "What they look for is that you feel bad so that you don't return." The following excerpts provide straightforward illustrations of the different effects:

CAROLINA: [I've been here for three hours now and] I won't be able to go to the soup kitchen today. They stop serving at noon, [if you want to eat] you have to arrive earlier.

INTERVIEWER: And you only applied for Nuestras Familias? Did you know that here they can help you with milk and diapers for your son?

C: Yes, I know, but I can't. I haven't asked for them because . . . *this is time*, and I can't ask permission everyday to come here . . . To have a subsidy you have to be here, be from here to there and from there to here. I need to work, necessity doesn't let me dedicate the time required for more subsidies. [my emphasis]

Two BAP social workers who, as we mentioned above, interact with the welfare office on a routine basis by bringing the homeless to apply for a housing subsidy, make candid remarks that summarize an all-too-common experience:

> "People get tired, it's like constant bad treatment. Not only in the interview, not just this waiting, it's the bad treatment. In a person whose situation is worse than any other person a priori, all of this is intensified. They have to wait two hours to be assisted, they have to wait two months to receive the subsidy. Officials then tell them something and later they tell them another thing [about the requirements]. They are all things that bother them, because one assumes that it would have to be a lot simpler, because in reality they aren't solving their lives. It is a brief subsidy that can help you a little, then it would have to be something extremely simple that doesn't complicate things. [At the welfare office] there is the idea that since they are poor, they have to wait . . ."

> "Obtaining a subsidy is tortuous. The process generates in people a tremendous tiredness, going to one office or another, reciting their problem three times. It is all an enormous debilitation."

The larger result of these delays and randomness is a seemingly contradictory process of both *bureaucratic disentitlement and snaring.* On the one hand, there is a constant reduction or elimination of benefits that takes place in the "hidden recesses of routine or obscure decision making" (Lipsky 1984: 3), such as the "eating up" of benefits described by a state agent and the pattern of "not every month" depicted by beneficiaries. On the other hand, in constantly asking beneficiaries to come back to check—an obligation that someone in need can hardly refuse— the state effectively *binds* the poor to the institution that is reducing both the benefits and their power.

This objective disorganization and bureaucratic indifference finds its subjective correlate in the experience of uncertainty and confusion. In writing about the nineteenth-century English proletariat, Friedrich Engels describes a class that "knows no security in life," a class that is a "playball to a thousand chances" (1973 [1844]: 139). Those waiting in the welfare office fit this description well. As detailed above, their lives are constantly "on the edge" of disaster or in the midst of it. They have recently been evicted or they are about to be, they have just lost their jobs, they are seriously sick, their spouses recently left them with three or more small children to be cared for and no stable source of household income, or they are dealing with any combination of the above. Once they come into the welfare waiting room, the insecurity does not stop.

Many of our subjects' descriptions of their waiting echo Engels's depiction of lives far away in time and place: "They kick us around like balls" (*Nos pelotean*). This simple statement captures the pervasive uncertainty and arbitrariness of the lived experience of waiting. The overwhelming majority of our subjects know when to come ("the earlier the better") to the office; most of them, however, don't know when they will leave. As Noemí laments while sitting in one of the few unoccupied chairs: "I told my husband: 'I'm going to the welfare office . . . don't know when I'm coming back.'" The following fieldnote and interview excerpts speak further about confusion and mistakes, endless delays, bureaucratic indifference, and the resulting peloteo as experienced by the dispossessed. We could easily interpret these interactions as instances of what Jeffry Prottas (1979) famously called "public degradation rituals":

November 11: The room is half full. Today, payments began earlier than usual. I meet Mabel and we are soon talking about her "situation."

MABEL: In the line they already warned me, because I asked a woman what it is I have to do and she warned me: "*Here, they are going to kick you around.*" [my emphasis]

INTERVIEWER: What happened to you?

M: They gave me a bad slip [to be attended to]. I waited an hour so that when they called me they told me that they couldn't help me there and that I had to get another slip again.

[She then tells in detail what they told her and where they sent her]

I: Who did you go to?

M: To that indifferent person over there [she shows me a young boy in a gray T-shirt, he isn't more than twenty-five].

I: Indifferent? Did he treat you badly?

M: Yes, badly. I gave him the slip and when he sees that it's bad he threw it back to me like this [she acts out the gesture by throwing an imaginary paper toward the place of the counter where she was standing].

In that moment an employee made her way to the room to call a group of people.

I: Did you hear her? I don't know what she said . . .

M: Nothing, she came to call the people who have the pink slip. They are herding them. [Referring to how the women start to wait standing, forming an unclear line close to the part of the reference desk at the counter, in the direction of the entrance of the building]

I: Herding?

M: But look, they crowd them there.

I: You aren't in these turns? Don't let your turn go because of me.

M: [going back to taking out the DNI from her purse and checking the number] Yes, yes, it's almost my turn. Better that I stand there to be attentive.

I: OK, go ahead. But Mabel, I have to stay another hour, so look for me when you leave so that you can tell me how it went, OK?

M: OK, yes, yes.

I: Good luck!

Mabel got up and walked in the direction of the counter. Her conversation with the employee lasted a little bit, but finally she withdrew herself from the counter. I had stopped watching her to take notes, and she called me by touching me on my back with her finger so that I returned my view to her. "They didn't want to assist me," she tells me. "Why? What did they tell you?" "That in order to begin the Nuestras Familias program I need a reference from a social worker." "But hadn't you precisely asked for an appointment with a social worker?" "But they didn't want to assist me . . ." . . . Mabel said goodbye, she didn't tell me if she would come back and I didn't ask either.

She was disillusioned. The only certainty was communicated to her by the other beneficiaries in the waiting room: Today they kicked her around.[2]

The interaction above also highlights the existence of two main types of waiters: those who know what to expect ("Here, you have to be patient") and those who do not, which coincides with the amount of time they have spent in the waiting room. First timers, like Mabel, are restless and impatient. They seek certainty and they assume that there are clearly established rules and protocols. Others—the majority— "know" what to expect when they come to the office; they know that much of what goes on is a game of chance and that they are at the mercy of state agents, and sometimes they communicate as much to the noninitiated.

The uncertainty about the amount of time they will spend in the office is combined with uncertainty about the outcome. *More than half (64 percent) of our eighty-nine interviewees do not know if or when they will receive the benefit they came to ask for.* This uncertainty does not vary by program, such as whether they are asking for a housing subsidy or food assistance, or by the citizenship status of the claimant. The "not knowing" is equally distributed among Argentine citizens and foreigners. The specific rules, regulations, and benefits of each welfare program do not seem to have an impact on the level of knowledge that people seem to have about their claims. This straightforward figure, however, cannot tell us much about the more interesting sociological phenomenon, namely the *protracted process* or *the web* that poor claimants have to traverse every time they need *urgent* aid. The following conversation takes place as Sofia and Hilda are awaiting a decision on two different welfare programs. Their doubts, their feelings, and the actual outcome of their petition vividly illustrate what I would call, following Pierre Bourdieu (2000), an "instituted disorder." As described below, this disorder is presented to the client as a result of the arbitrary dictums of a computer.

December 11, 2008: Sofía, in her early thirties, moved to Argentina from Paraguay in 1999. She first came to the welfare office when she was evicted from her rental apartment. Hilda is twenty-eight and moved from Paraguay in 1998. When her husband left her, she quickly ran out of money to pay for the rent—she was about to be evicted when a neighborhood social worker told her to come to the office. With two small kids, she is having trouble finding a place to live—"hotels won't take you with children," she tells me, echoing what we heard repeatedly from poor mothers who are raising their kids alone.

Sofía and Hilda have been at the welfare office for forty minutes already when I meet them. Sofía addresses the issue of the long waiting right from the start: "You can be here for three or four hours." "Why?" I ask. "That's exactly what we'd like to know: why do we have to wait that long? Afterward, they tell you there's no money and that you have to come back some other day." Sofía began her paperwork for the Nuestras Familias five months ago. She received her first check this week but she was expecting a sum three times higher, "They suspended my payments three times already. Supposedly, I'll get paid today." She is also a beneficiary of the Subsidio Habitacional, but she says that she is "not being paid. I don't know what's going on." Someone at the counter calls Sofía. She leaves. Like Sofía, Hilda does not know if and when she will receive her check: "Last year, I didn't get paid. They told me 'We can't do anything about it . . . [they say] it is what it is.'"

Sofía comes back and tells me that her payment was suspended again. "They told me to come back on December 30. I've been waiting since July. I don't know what we're going to do. That's what pisses me off."

We then talk about the required paperwork and they agree that it is "too difficult": "They always give you an excuse. . . . They ask you for some document, then they ask for it again and again, and you have to come back at 5 AM. . . . Now they are attending quickly, but there's no money. Damn."

Both of them have come to this office many times before. And many times they have been "rescheduled," which is the term used by state agents and beneficiaries alike to describe the delay in the payments. It is now Hilda's turn. She goes to the counter and quickly comes back. She is also "rescheduled." "They told me that there is only one payment left. Originally, there were four, but now it's only one. I don't know why. *That's what the computer says*" [emphasis added].

The welfare recipients described by Sharon Hays complain primarily about the hassles to obtain welfare, and like some of the beneficiaries we encountered they point to the "huge number of ridiculous regulations" (2003: 7) that make their already-miserable life even more wretched. Hays describes the universe of welfare reform in the United States as a place where there are confusions, misunderstandings, and frustrations with the rules, requirements, procedures, and sanctions, and her description finds parallels in the world of Buenos Aires welfare. However, for people like Sofía, Hilda, and many others, the main issues are not so much the paperwork or requirements but the *unpredictability* of the process. Some of them complain about the "difficult paperwork," but what really bothers most of them is the long waiting period and its insecure results. As twenty-three-year-old Isabel, who migrated from Peru two years ago and who is waiting for the Nuestras Familias payments, stated succinctly: "You don't know when you are going to be paid."

More than half of our interviewees used the experience of *waiting in a public hospital* to compare and contrast it with the welfare office. Although they all agreed that waiting in the hospital is "terrible," "awful," and they remark that they "always" have to wait there, they also know, as Isabel comments, that in a hospital "they will attend you no matter what." Both waiting lines, they all concur, are long ("you can spend the entire day at the hospital"); both waiting times demand their endurance and serenity ("we all know how it is"; "there is not much you can do about it"). The hospital line is, to most, "more dramatic," because they usually attend the hospital when they are seriously sick or when their children need immediate assistance. By contrast, "here [in the welfare office] the waiting is *indecisa* [indecisive]." Isabel's statement captures well the randomness of the entire process: "I think I'll be paid . . . at Christmas, which is when miracles occur."

As stated above, uncertainty is neither restricted to noncitizens nor to the admission stage; rather, it characterizes the operation of the office as a whole. Noemí is a fifty-five-year-old Argentine citizen, and she tells us that she is in the office "because of an administrative error, they delayed my payment for a week . . . plus the three or four hours of waiting here." Apparently, mistakes are not the only source of intermittence in the welfare payments. In Noemí's experience, as with most of the beneficiaries we interviewed, haphazardness is a built-in characteristic of city welfare programs. Once clients are admitted, in other words, their payments can be suspended or delayed for reasons unknown to them: "If the hotel owners were not merciful, they would kick us out because . . . well, nobody tells you when you are going to be paid. They [welfare agents] tell you it's going to be on the fifth and they pay you on the fourteenth." Noemí is also the beneficiary of another welfare program, a cash transfer program that is equally random: "Every month they put money in your account for you to spend. Well, it's a way of putting it. Sometimes it is every forty days. Do you know how shameful you feel when you go to the supermarket, you buy all this stuff, and then you have to leave it there with the cashier because your [welfare] card has no funds?!"

"They tell you one thing, and then another," said Rosa angrily. She is a forty-five-year-old woman who is petitioning for a housing subsidy, and she was summarizing for us what goes on in the welfare office. Rosa ended our hour-long conversation crying, saying, "I'm a grown-up person, and they tell me [come] tomorrow, [come] tomorrow, [come] tomorrow." Probably the most straightforward illustration of the lived uncertainty was the innumerable times we heard clients asking each other (and us): "Do you know if they are paying today?" Or, as was often repeated out loud: "Nobody knows anything here."

Along with their perceptions of uncertainty and confusion, most welfare clients articulate feelings of despondency and futility. There is a reason for these feelings, and it is not in the poor people's "value system" or in any other durable "cultural" trait they might have. The feeling of dejection and inadequacy is context specific ("You feel impotent *here*") and stems from their own inability to influence the workings of the welfare office ("There's not much you can do, you have to wait"). In writing about the self-efficacy mechanism in human agency, Albert Bandura distinguishes two sources of perceived uselessness:

"People can give up trying because they seriously doubt that they can do what is required. Or they may be assured of their capabilities but give up trying because they expect their efforts to produce no results due to the *unresponsiveness, negative bias, or punitiveness of the environment*" (1982: 140; my emphasis). Welfare clients do not have many options; they cannot "exit," to use Albert Hirschman's now famous expression. So they continue to try, they keep coming. They don't publicly "voice" much of their discontent, as I will show in more detail below, because their sense of agency is infused by a perceived ineffectiveness. They simply don't think that protest can make much of a difference. We could then hypothesize, drawing upon the insights of social cognitive theory, that the very uncertain and arbitrary operation of the welfare office produces what, to borrow from Bandura, is an "outcome-based (perceived) futility" (1982: 140).

THE FETISHISM OF THE BENEFIT

The following dialogue, recorded as we were seeking permission to conduct our fieldwork, describes a typical interaction between a state agent and a claimant. The interaction was typical in that the agent was cordial but the outcome was undefined. It is also typical of the issue of extreme depersonalization, in that the computer system is presented as the one responsible for scheduling the payments. No human actor is deemed accountable for delays and suspensions. Despite the official's polite handling of the case, the reasons for the rescheduling always remain obscure. Since the only one who really "knows" when the payment will be made is the computer (or "the system"), complaints and negotiations are precluded. Rescheduling is automatic and not open to appeal.

September 18, 2008:
STATE AGENT (SA) [referring to the program Nuestras Familias]:
   Did you ever get paid?
BENEFICIARY (B): No, because I had my baby and couldn't come
   because he was too little . . .

SA: [interrupting]: You are Gutierrez, aren't you?

B: [nods, affirmatively]

SA: You never got paid . . . The system reprograms the installments
    by itself. You have to come back on October 2. You will then
    have two installments ready to be paid. For the time being
    everything is suspended, but come anyway. . . .

The reason I cite this seemingly trivial interaction is the fact that the
payment postponements were continuously *justified in terms of the
pronouncements made by the computer.* The payments are "reprogrammed," and so are the welfare beneficiaries. "You've been reprogrammed," state agents tell clients. "I've been reprogrammed," subjects
echoed. In this way, the "mystical veil" (Marx 1887: 84) of the computer program ends up disguising the politics of welfare. The actual
administration of benefits remains a "secret, hidden under the apparent fluctuations" (77) of a software program. The social and political
relations between citizens and the state at the basis of welfare assume
"the fantastic form" of a relation between a check and a computer. As
the following excerpts illustrate, the fetishism of the benefit remains
suspended in doubt and confusion throughout the time the client is
eligible for welfare.

September 18, 2008: The state agent is looking at the computer screen and
talking to (but not facing) the welfare client: "Your next payday is October 9.
You were paid September. August is delayed and it has to be reprogrammed.
In order to be reprogrammed, come on the ninth. You will be paid October
and we will reprogram you then." The client nods and leaves.

INTERVIEWER: And how did you find out about this place?

OLINDA: From acquaintances who told me: "Go there and they will help
you."

I: And how long ago did you start the procedure of the Nuestras Familias?

O: Since quite a while already . . . yes it's already quite a while. One time
   they told me to come and when I came they told me that they aren't
   going to give it to me, that it still isn't approved, that I return in three
   weeks again. I returned again and they told me that I didn't appear in

the system. They told me that the process still wasn't appearing in the computer, another time that they aren't going to pay, that I come back, and like that . . . Another time I came again and they told me that it was ready but that I have to return to confirm the payment date . . .

I: Then you have come three times only to see if they had accepted you yet . . .

O: Three times . . . no! More, many more times.

I: When did you first come?

O: The first time was last year, but I did the procedure and they only paid me two times, then it was a new year and they told me that I had to return to renew.

I: Did you renew?

O: No . . .

I: And why did they tell you that you have to renew?

O: I don't know because they only paid me twice and there are six installments.

INTERVIEWER: How long ago did you start the procedure of the Nuestras Familias?

NANCY: A long time ago. In July I started the procedure. And today [early December] is going to be the first day that I collect [my payment].

I: Since July until today?

N: Yes.

I: And what explanations did they give you for not giving it to you earlier?

N: At first they told me that I didn't appear in the system, that I [need to] return the following week. I returned and since I continued to not be in the system they told me to return the following week, or at the end of the month.

I: Did they always tell you that?

N: Later they told me that I was accepted but that they couldn't give me a date because the deposit wasn't ready. The men over there [the agents at the counter] told me, "I don't know what's up, I don't have anything to do with it, the money doesn't arrive because the deposit isn't there."

I: How many times per month did you come?

N: Three at the minimum. Sometimes I also called on the phone. There is

a telephone where you can find out, did you see? I called and they told
me, "No ma'am, you don't show up in the system."

I: And you never protested?

N: Protest, protest . . . no. But I did ask how it is that women who I knew
that had started in September or October already received [payment]
and I, who started in July, still didn't receive anything . . .

I: [interrupting her] . . . and did they answer you?

N: . . . what I told you, they told me that the deposit isn't there, that I am
accepted but the money hasn't arrived . . .

In many other fieldnotes, we also recorded welfare agents telling
clients things along the following lines: "Everything is delayed; you
have to come back next week to see if there is news"; "No, no . . . it's all
suspended, you have to come back next week and find out." These
discursive interactions, or what we could call pronouncements, depict
welfare distribution as a "mysterious thing" (akin to Marx's commodity); and yet they also portray the *demands that the state makes to the
claimants.* Keep coming, the agents implicitly or explicitly tell the beneficiaries. Neither we nor you know when you will receive the actual
welfare payment, but you have to keep coming. The state, through its
authorized spokespersons, tells the poor that if they want a successful
resolution of their claim, they have to wait. For how long? They are
never told. Two more examples, heard countless times by us and by the
clients, should suffice to depict the constant deferrals and delays, the
veritable exercising of power over poor people's time, to which welfare
clients are routinely exposed: "Everything is late today, you have to
come back next week to see if there is any news"; "Your next payday is
November 25. You should not miss that day because you are going to be
paid for September. We'll then see . . ."

SIT DOWN AND WAIT

Poor people come to this same welfare room to ask about the same
welfare program or about the same overdue installments several times
during the course of the year. Most of those we talked to said they had

come to this office on more than one occasion to claim for the same benefit or to see if the same cash installment was finally ready. Given the random changes described above, the recurrent "reprogramming," and the constant delays and cancellations, clients *must* come to the office on a regular basis. Welfare clients are thus frequent visitors of the waiting room. Given this recursive exposure and the particular relationship to the state that is hammered in the hearts and minds of the poor, the welfare office should be thought of not simply as a "people processing" institution (Hasenfeld 1972) but as a "people changing" operation (see Comfort 2008); that is, a patterned set of interactions with concrete subjective effects.

In contrast to other places where bad information and uncertainty produce a "bargaining process" between those who know and those who do not (Goffman 1961; Roth 1963), the waiting room is defined as an area of compliance, a universe where you "sit down and wait" instead of attempting to negotiate with or complain against welfare authorities. When asked, more than a third of our interviewees have negative comments about welfare agents. Most of them grumble about occasional mistreatments. However, in *the regular course of the waiting* these complaints are muted. Only three times during our twelve months of fieldwork did we witness clients addressing state agents with complaints out loud.

Jorge is a recipient of a Nuestras Familias benefit and is currently applying to the housing subsidy. Using language echoed by many others, he describes the long delays involved in both programs. When asked what he does when confronted with these delays, his response was a familiar one; it was what another beneficiary described as "simply asking, nothing more, not complaining really." The state tells people like Jorge that, since they are in need, their time has no value. They will have to wait, which means to endure long delays and to put up with *malos tratos* (bad treatment). Jorge and most of the others we interacted with heed the state's commands, believing that if they are in real need they have to put up with the state's bad treatment and lengthy, unpredictable schedule.

INTERVIEWER: What do you do when they delay the payment?

JORGE: *Nothing. I wait. I don't make a mess or a racket*, because I need it and they are the ones who are going to pay me anyway. And it's true, it's hard, one shouldn't let that happen . . . I even know people who don't want the help because they dislike the way in which they are treated; [they say], "No, no, I already went two months, there they treat you bad and I prefer not to know about the place anymore." *But it's like that, if you are in need you have to wait.*" [my emphasis]

In none of our eighty-nine interviews did current and prospective beneficiaries refer to themselves as "patients." María alone used the term "patient" to refer to people like her. Although the word is unique, it describes well the process that most (if not all) have to go through.

MARÍA: They delay attending to you. They don't listen to you, they are there but they don't listen to you.

INTERVIEWER: They don't pay attention to you?

M: I don't know if they are eating breakfast, until 10 they eat breakfast, drink mate, [eat] cookies; they talk a lot among themselves.

I: And how do you get their attention?

M: No, I wait for them to assist me.

I: You just wait for them to pay attention to you?

M: It's that you just have to wait.

I: Of all the times that you have gone, do you remember if there was any time a commotion was made there?

M: One time yes [she laughs a little] . . . with a social worker.

I: What happened?

M: I don't know well, but a *patient* fought shouting with the social worker, until she said something to her that made them fight with their hands.

I: What patient, some kind of health patient?

M: No, *a patient here, a woman who waited.* [my emphasis]

The overall lack of contention over what is for us as observers a rather grievous process should not be seen as passivity on the part of welfare recipients and applicants. In fact, we have plenty of evidence to the contrary. Poor people are actively seeking solutions to their problems and they strategize accordingly.[3] The following fieldnote excerpt summarizes this constant maneuvering:

> *September 25, 2009*: Before I was able to describe the purpose of my visit, Cebelina and Claudio were the most willing to help me in my first day of visiting. Carlos asked me if I was there for a housing subsidy and starts to throw at me the list of requirements and the procedure that I have to follow immediately. "Look, to apply to the subsidy you have to demonstrate that you are homeless or that you can't pay the place where you are staying. Once you fill out the process form a lady is going to visit you the next day and is going to corroborate what you said before. If they approve you after that you are ready. . . . Are you renting anywhere? Bring a payment receipt . . . if you can talk with the landlady and ask her to put a little more than what it costs you in reality. . . . They don't give you more than 450 pesos for six months, although then you can extend it for four more months. The payment doesn't suffice, but it helps, you finish with a peso here, a peso there."

Active problem-solving should not, however, be confused with resistance to the dreadful process of waiting.[4] We found neither hidden transcripts (Scott 1990) nor open contestation to the dominant understanding of time at the welfare office. Occasionally, people complain by implicitly asserting that the office should operate otherwise, and they direct the blame for the delays against "slob" agents who "take too many breaks," "who don't care," "who don't want to work," and "who have breakfast until 10 AM," to quote the most common expressions. Other times, they blame not the "lazy" state agents but those who do not deserve welfare benefits, those who, to quote an often-heard assertion, "do not need because they have a business, or a job." According to many, these "undeserving" clients, "those who don't need but come and collect," overburden the welfare rolls and make them wait longer. As with every act of blaming, this one invokes some standard of justice (Tilly 2008). As Milagros (whose story opened the previous chapter) put it: "There's people here who don't need. That's not fair. They have their own business." The statement is relevant not because it describes the welfare population we studied (we do not have evidence to back up those who believe that there are many people with good and stable incomes among the clients) but because it points to the *self-understanding* of the welfare population (Brubaker and Cooper 2000) and to a *symbolic boundary* (Lamont and Molnar 2002) that organizes the experience of waiting. Most of the people we talked to and observed think of themselves as a population in "need." They come to the welfare office not because they have a "right"—in hundreds of pages of fieldnotes and interviews, the word "right" does not appear once—but because they are "in need." Those who do not need but who apply and obtain welfare benefits and therefore "take advantage" are perceived as the cause of the long waiting lines.

"It's an aid," we heard repeatedly. That is how welfare clients "in need" understand their benefits; again, not as "rights" but as "aid" or "help." "And sometimes they help you and sometimes they don't," they frequently say. "Those in need" come to the welfare office and are faced with the general disorganization and disinformation described above, along with the endless delays and also with the sudden rushing of surprise paydays, and therefore they quickly learn that this is a space to be a complying welfare client. They learn that if they want the benefit they have to yield to the arbitrary, uncertain wishes or dictates of state agents and of machines. They know that they have to remain in expectation and to comply with the random operation of the welfare office. As Ramiro told us while he waited for three long hours, leaning against the wall: "You can't complain here, if you do, they send you back home . . . So, you have to stay calm here." Or, as many others stated: "Here, you have to be patient . . . you have to arm yourself with patience." Milagros summarized it well by saying, "Here, I didn't say anything"; that is, she did not voice her discontent. The recurrent comparison that welfare clients make between their waiting time at public hospitals and their time at the welfare office thus takes on its full meaning. In both places they have to silently endure and act not as citizens with rightful claims but as patients of the state.

To analyze waiting is arduous for two reasons. The first is because of the absence of much activity to be observed and recorded; and the second, and most important, is because waiting—and especially the waiting of the materially and symbolically dispossessed—is invested with the "objectivity of a common sense, a practical, doxic consensus on the sense of practices" (Bourdieu 2001: 33), much like masculine domination. Everybody—including state officials, social workers, and the poor themselves—thinks of the waiting of the destitute as something obvious and unavoidable. Some recipients even believe it is necessary: "If you want to receive the benefit, you need to wait."

The mundane daily operation of this office and the seemingly ordinary assertions of state agents and clients jointly—but hardly cooperatively—defines what we could call the *doxa of welfare* (Bourdieu 1998). This is a basic agreement, for the most part uncontested, on the fundamental presuppositions of welfare distribution: Show patience, wait, and you might obtain a benefit from the state. Suggestions ("Come back tomorrow and we'll see what we can do"), injunctions ("You've been reprogrammed"), and calls to order ("All of you, form a line against the wall") could thus be understood as expressions of symbolic violence. These expressions exercise their power by working through acts of knowledge and practical recognition on the part of the dominated. People in the waiting room know that they have to come back several times to obtain a positive response, they know that they have to demonstrate endurance and worth to state agents, and they know they have to wait because, as Mario who is awaiting a decision on a housing subsidy so eloquently put it, "in this country, waiting is a classic, you live in the waiting [*uno vive en la espera*]."

THE FEMALE PATIENT:

STRUCTURING GENDER AT THE WELFARE OFFICE

Norita was born in Paraguay and has been living in Buenos Aires for
more than ten years. The unreliability and unpredictability of the welfare office and the wearing-down effect of long delays come together in
her testimony. Yet once we place her story in the context of existing
welfare policies (the programs, their objectives, and their target populations), another key dimension emerges, that of gender. Norita was
receiving the housing subsidy when she suddenly stopped receiving
payments.

> INTERVIEWER: And why did they stop giving it to you?
> NORITA: I don't know. They gave me two payments, and then they
>   put up obstacles. One day they just told me that the payment
>   for foreigners still hadn't been resolved.
> I: And what did you do then to know when they were going to
>   pay you or when they weren't?
> N: Oh, then they get you coming every week to ask, because here
>   nobody calls to you to say "the payment is ready."
> I: And what did you do with that uncertainty in order to get to
>   the end of the month?
> N: No, it's that I luckily don't depend on that. My husband works
>   and I do too. Listen, *if you depend on that to live, you are on the
>   street . . .* [my emphasis]. It helps me, it's of service to me, but I
>   don't rely on it, thank God. I would be on the street.
> I: And what did you do when they told you that they weren't
>   going to keep paying you?
> N: They never told me that they weren't going to pay me more,
>   only that they still hadn't resolved the payment for foreigners. I
>   came and I came. For two months I was coming, until I grew
>   tired. Then I applied to the Nuestras Familias.

Needless to say, and not surprisingly, the welfare waiting room is a
space dominated by women. The four main welfare programs target
women, either explicitly by formally restricting access to women only

or implicitly by in practice granting benefits mostly to women. In other words, the patient of the state that is being manufactured at the welfare office is primarily a female patient. What are the implications of this fact?

The language of the Ministerio de Desarrollo Social, as articulated in its official publications,[5] is genderless, and it speaks about its attempt to "include . . . excluded citizens," and of "assisting" and "socially promoting" the "most vulnerable" families and individuals. Nevertheless, the "target population" of its focalized programs is overwhelmingly female. Note, for example, that as of November 2009, 89.3 percent of the beneficiaries of the cash transfer program (Ciudadania Porteña) are women.[6] The Ticket Social, which is another cash transfer program that provides a monthly check of US$25 that can be used to purchase food and cleaning and sanitary products, is restricted to women only.

Most of the people we waited with were expecting resolutions or payments from two other programs (the Nuestras Familias and the Subsidio Habitacional) administered by the Dirección General de Asistencia Inmediata, though as we saw, there is nothing "immediate" in the operation of this agency. Although formally open to everybody, these two programs also focus mainly on women. Among the objectives of the housing subsidy is to provide assistance to the families who are in *situación de calle*—or homeless, to use a less euphemistic term— by "strengthening the family income" that is devoted to paying for shelter.[7] Although the target population of the benefit is "the family," the first requirement points to the household composition, with special consideration given to "female-headed families." Although not explicitly articulated in official documents, a similar gender bias affects the Nuestras Familias. Among its objectives is to "strengthen family groups" who are in "vulnerable situations" or at "risk of not being able to satisfy their basic needs." In practice, however, women are again the main target. As an official of the welfare agency told us: "It is difficult for men to obtain benefits. Because there's the idea that if a man is at a working age, he has to work. More benefits are given to mothers." This gendered conception is further reinforced by the Ministerio's policies toward men. In the section of the Ministerio's social services guide

describing the "strategic objectives" for 2010, we read that the agency
seeks to: "1. Increase social inclusion and strengthen equal opportu-
nities for the most vulnerable groups; 2. Increase employment among
vulnerable *fathers* [my emphasis]." Under the first point, the Ministerio's policies will pay "special attention" to the issue of violence
against women with "lectures, workshops, treatment, and seminars."
Under the second point, they will "double the amount of job training
fellowships for vulnerable fathers."

As we detected in the waiting room and now see articulated in
official documents, welfare is structured around women. For them, the
state provides limited and random welfare benefits such as shelter,
food, and protection against violence. For men, it seeks to provide
access to full employment. This represents a gender pattern that re-
produces the bifurcation within the welfare state of male independent
workers and female dependent non-workers (Pateman 1988; Orloff
1993; Fraser 1989; Gordon 1990a; Haney 1996). Men are conceived of
as subjects who rely on the labor market, while women are constructed
as submissive clients of the state.

Welfare programs structure gender relations in yet another way. In
adapting the work of socialist feminists on the state's enforcement of
patriarchal social order (Gordon 1990a, 1990b), we could also argue
that the state—and in particular the welfare office—*encourages* female
dependence. By making shelter inaccessible and by keeping welfare
payments meager, the state implicitly coerces women to attach themselves to male breadwinners who can provide either housing or more
stable sources of income. Norita's statement and the many others that
we heard about the insufficiency and unreliability of the welfare funds
("You can't depend on this"; "If you depend on this you'd be [living]
on the street"; "If you depend on this, you are dead") now take an
additional meaning. The state seems to be telling women not only that
they should be patient but also that if they rely on welfare funds to
make ends meet they would also have to depend on their husbands or
male partners for food and shelter. At the level of *welfare practice*,
therefore, the state upholds private patriarchy—the reliance of individual women on individual men.

We therefore see that at the level of daily practice the state is doing more than simply reproducing a particular kind of relationship with the poor. The daily work of the state is structured around gender differences and in turn structures gender hierarchy (see Mink 1990; Nelson 1990).[8]

Germán Solioz had lung cancer. He died in August 1998 after having stayed in an intensive care unit for a month and a half. Two years before her father's death, Gladys Solioz cut out from a scientific journal an article that warned about the danger of high-tension electrical wiring in urban areas. "They are coming here," she thought, and put the page away. There was a small warehouse of the state-owned electricity company Servicios Eléctricos del Gran Buenos Aires (SEGBA) next to her house. The Municipality of Quilmes assured that it would be converted to a square, the same as the one where Gladys remembers playing when she lived half a block away. But so far the square is just a memory from childhood. Had Gladys and her husband known that the true designation of the land on the corner would be otherwise, they would not have started building the face-brick house where they now live at the age of forty-five with their three children. After the privatization of the company (it is now called Empresa Distribuidora Sur Sociedad Anónima [EDESUR]), workers arrived one September morning in 1992. Gladys's clipping folder kept on growing as thick as a telephone directory of a big city. It contains the medical histories and death certificates of most of the nearly two thousand neighbors who live in the eleven blocks around her house. There is also a map inside the folder; a sketch that Gladys has been making by hand for several years. When unfolded, the sketch occupies half of the dining room table. On it, she draws green crosses indicating neighbors suffering from cancer. The red crosses are dedicated to those who passed away. It is ten years now since she started the home-made census and the count comes to 115 dead and 112 ill.[1]

The case of Gladys and her neighbors is sadly familiar. Engaging in a version of "popular epidemiology" (Brown and Mikkelsen 1990), Gladys has been creating a map that records sickness and death (see fig. 6). Cases of leukemia, breast cancer, colon cancer, and lung cancer abound in the eleven-block area surrounding her home, all presumably the result of the powerful electromagnetic field generated by Subestación Sobral, a power-transformer plant located in Ezpeleta, which is a half-hour drive from downtown Buenos Aires in the district of Quilmes. The plant receives 132,000 volts and distributes 220 volts, from which it provides electricity to the populous districts of Quilmes and Avellaneda. Gladys's house sits adjacent to the substation.

Yet Gladys is not merely a witness of collective suffering. As a sort of Argentine Erin Brockovich, she has also been leading the struggle to close and move the plant. The decade-and-a-half long protest has included blocking with their own bodies and those of their little children the construction of concrete pillars to support the high voltage wires coming out from the power plant, a variety of collective actions against EDESUR's initiatives, and even meetings with the company's regional CEO.

After being diagnosed with cancer in 1999, Angélica Boncosqui joined her neighbor Gladys in what they call *la lucha* (the struggle) against EDESUR's power plant (see fig. 7). Since then, they have been inseparable friends. Together, they met with affected neighbors, lawyers, and state officials. It has not been an easy task. As they told us when we interviewed them in July 2010, neighbors are "hard to persuade. They don't want to talk about cancer."[2] According to them, state officials such as the ombudsman tell them that "it's a big problem. Reason is on your side, but we don't know how to solve it"; and until recently, lawyers "did not want to take up the case because they said it's a very powerful transnational company" or, worse, they "ended up making *arreglos* [under-the-table deals]" with the company.

Angélica and Gladys's activism does not stop in Ezpeleta. They also join other protests against similar power plants in neighboring towns, such as the one in nearby Berazategui. They see their activism as a form

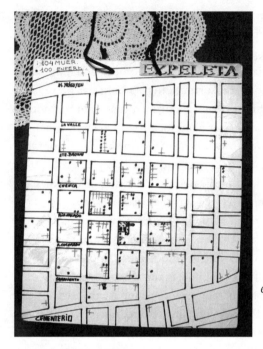

6 Map of death in
Ezpeleta. Courtesy
of Agustín Burbano
de Lara.

of "consciousness-raising" so that others "don't have to go through
what we are going through." And they take pride in their unwavering
fight against what they both perceive as mighty interests. As Gladys
told us: "If, God forbids, I ever get cancer, I know I will not regret what
I've done. I'm proud of this struggle. Because if I get sick I'll know that
I did everything I could."

In the early stages of their protest, they counted on the support of a
few local politicians. As time went by and their struggle and determi-
nation deepened, they felt that politicians began to take the side of
their opposition, the company: "At the beginning we felt he [the coun-
cilman] was closer to us." In their minds, the reason for this distance is
clear: the company buys people out, not only politicians but also journalists, lawyers, scientists, and even neighbors, as the following comments show: "Once the local newspaper did a report on the neighborhood, and then, a few days later, a big advertisement paid by EDESUR

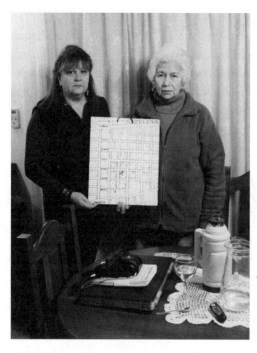

7 Gladys (left) and
Angélica holding the
map of Ezpeleta.
Courtesy of Agustín
Burbano de Lara.

was published in the newspaper, and the report never came out";
"EDESUR hires experts to invalidate our claims and to deny the deaths
and the sickness that is all around us." According to Angélica and
Gladys, one of the first leaders of the protest accepted money from
EDESUR, and other neighbors received goods in exchange for their silence. "The company buys [everybody's] silence," they suspect. "More
than once, journalists told us that we were banned in the local paper . . .
banned by the company." As I stated in *Flammable: Environmental
Suffering in an Argentine Shantytown*, the book I wrote with Débora
Swistun in 2009, I believe that even when we cannot corroborate their
veracity, these suspicions and stories should be taken seriously because
they are an essential part of living in a dangerous place. In the analysis
of environmental suffering and "toxic waiting," the issue is not what a
company, a state official, a journalist, a scientist, or a lawyer really are or
do but how they are perceived to be and to behave.

In 2003, in response to a lawsuit that Gladys, Angélica, and a few neighbors had initiated with the help of lawyers from the Asamblea Permanente de Derechos Humanos (APDH), a court order was made to stop the enlargement of the plant. Despite the fact that the order arrived late, and the planned improvements of the plant's capacity had already been done, the lawsuit was successful in raising the neighbors' expectations about possibility of the plant's relocation (*Clarín*, July 17, 2003; *Página12*, July 16, 2003). "That is what we want," Gladys told us, "the plant's relocation." "If this were a soccer match," another neighbor stated, "we could compare this court order to having won the first half. We still need to win the match—that is, the relocation of the plant to a place where nobody is living close to it" (*Clarín*, July 17, 2003). It has been, however, a very long second half; since the 2003 court order nothing has happened. Neighbors are still living, suffering, and dying close to Subestación Sobral.[3] As Gladys told a journalist from *Perfil* in an article published on June 6, 2009: "We have made presentations to the court that sought a quick resolution . . . something like a *recurso de amparo* [writ of protection].[4] We made a presentation in 2002 and it's now 2009 and we are still waiting for the judge to evaluate the situation and to decide on the relocation of the substation." Gladys is here referring to one of the judicial claims that residents affected by environmental hazards have at their disposal according to Argentine law. It is a legal claim of termination that mandates the immediate cessation of the activity causing environmental damage (the other being the legal claim of reparation) (Kohen et al. 2001). According to Argentine law and jurisprudence, this type of legal claim should be handled through *amparos* (summary trials) and may require *medidas cautelares* (precautionary measures). These measures, ordered by the courts, aim at the immediate cessation of the acts or omissions that are causing damage. For this measure to thrive, claimants need to verify the *periculum in mora* (the danger in the delay).

"Our time is not the time of the one who has to solve the problem. Ours is a particular, special time. Because the sick person's time is not the judge's time. He [the judge] is the one who has to decide the relocation of the power plant; that's what we are asking for. I have cancer, my time is different, my urgency is different. It's about my life," Angélica told us. Gladys made the following, more specific, statement regarding different temporal horizons by sketching what she believes is the modus operandi of the justice system and of EDESUR's delaying maneuverings: "EDESUR is always obstructing the judge's orders. They answer the court's requests with thousands of documents. When the judge finishes reading them, it'll be the year 3000. It is as if EDESUR is using up time, so that the process lasts forever, and we give up. I think EDESUR might be waiting [i.e., expecting] until Angélica dies and I get sick." Gladys and Angélica know that a prolonged waiting time is ahead of them: "It is as if the court case is stuck now. It's a file that is too heavy, too 'hot,' so to speak, with a lot of lawyers involved." They also think the company is engaged in another more pernicious form of waiting: EDESUR is, they both believe, awaiting the protest's demise, either in the form of a resigned surrender, a "throwing in the towel" of sorts, or in the form of the protesters' physical disappearance.

The case of Ezpeleta is a stark example of the peril that thousands of people exposed to environmental hazards are forced to endure. Despite the "danger in the delay" that is obvious to anybody who cares to look at Gladys's map, the sluggish reactions of courts and state officials impose an endless waiting time on weak, sick, and powerless residents. This waiting is occasionally interrupted by orders and initiatives, whose only real outcome is to raise collective hopes that are then silently crushed by the passing of time. In what follows, I examine another case of waiting in the midst of toxic assault as I focus on the role that state agents play in the production of *meaningful waiting*. I also indirectly illuminate the investment that endangered citizens make in the outcome of long-expected decisions.

BACK IN FLAMMABLE

The Buenos Aires suburb of Flammable is a highly contaminated neighborhood adjacent to a petrochemical compound, an unmonitored landfill, a hazardous waste incinerator, and a polluted river where I conducted ethnographic fieldwork five years ago. I begin this revisit by paraphrasing the opening scene of Kafka's *The Trial*. Someone must have slandered the neighborhood's residents, because one morning, without having done anything wrong, they find themselves waiting. They are waiting to be relocated or evicted; waiting for the results of a new blood or urine test that would let them know whether or not they are "contaminated" (*para saber si estamos o no contaminados*); and waiting for the courts to rule on a lawsuit that would grant them a dreamed indemnification for health damages. Much like Vladimir and Estragon, they are not waiting alone. And similar to Josef K.'s case, the waiting is interrupted by officials' routinely renewed promises and lawyers' sporadic references to progress. Unlike Josef K., however, this process is also interspersed with occasional distributions of concrete benefits, such as new homes for a few selected residents. These rewards demonstrate to the neighbors left behind that their waiting is not totally "in vain," thus further ensnaring them in the waiting process.

I return here to Flammable to chronicle some of the events that took place since the publication of *Flammable* in 2009. A few changes have occurred in the neighborhood, and one of the families of the original study, along with two dozen others, were relocated to a new housing complex. However, the general state of the barrio's dwellers is the same, which is summarized in the words of one old-timer: "We are still waiting." This experience of waiting, I will show in this final chapter, dovetails with a certain experience of politics.

After "engaging" his lawyer, Josef K. keeps "waiting expectantly for (him) to take action." Like K., Flammable residents are "lured" with vague hopes (an indemnification, a new home) and "tormented" with unclear threats (eviction is always "about to happen"). Like him, they continue to wait for someone to take action on their behalf. In what follows I will reconstruct their points of view on waiting and on politics, and present evidence that attests to their mutual imbrication in the schemes of thought held by residents. In drawing upon the in-depth interviews conducted for the original study (in 2004 and 2005) and the new interviews carried out in 2009 and 2010, I will argue that both waiting and politics are lived as profoundly disempowering processes. These two lived experiences tend to reinforce each other, generating the shared perception that the motor or the initiative of transformative action lies elsewhere. From these reconstructions of the residents' point of view, real outcomes are not and could not be generated by them. Rather, outcomes are determined by those who, in the residents' own words, seldom "come down" to the neighborhood. Politics, that "thing" that takes place "up there," determines their fate. This shared understanding is typical among residents in other neighborhoods of relegation in contemporary Buenos Aires, and it is one key effect of domination. Most people we talked to do not see themselves as agents capable of modifying their own conditions of existence, which are in Flammable's case highly polluted.

Let me return to Flavia Bellomi's fieldnotes in chapter 2 on the daily life of elementary schoolchildren in a poor enclave. On June 9, 2009, she noted that one of her students, Manuel, has been missing for many days. Her mother came to tell her that, just like her other children, Manuel is "full of pimples." These are skin rashes most likely produced by the family's location on the banks of the Riachuelo, the highly contaminated river that divides the city of Buenos Aires from the southern suburbs.[5] Close to five million people live in the Matanza-Riachuelo river basin, and 35 percent of them lack potable water, 60 percent do not have sewage systems, and 10 percent live in precarious settlements close to open-air garbage-dumping sites.

Following the course of the Riachuelo north and east, tons of toxic sludge, diluted solvents, lead, and cadmium, are all routinely tossed into the river's dead stream by meat-packing plants, chemical industries, tanneries, and households. It is no coincidence that this river has been defined by the federal ombudsman as "the worst ecological disaster of the country" (*Clarín*, May 12, 2003). Furthermore a significant proportion of the massive shantytown growth in Buenos Aires has taken place along its banks, and at least thirteen *villas miseria* (shantytowns) are located adjacent to it.

Where the Riachuelo meets the Río de la Plata is one of the largest petrochemical compounds in the country, and it is the site of Shell Oil

Corporation's only oil refinery in the Southern Cone. The shantytown of Flammable (its real name is Villa Inflamable) is located directly across from the compound. The images in figures 8–12 were taken by the neighborhood's elementary schoolchildren in a photography workshop we organized in the second semester of 2009, and they portray a few of the residents' homes, the barrio's general landscape, and the compound's smokestacks as seen from Flammable.[6] As reported in our original study, shantytown children still see themselves as living in the "midst of garbage and poison."

The Shell-Capsa oil refinery is the most important plant in the area, but the compound also houses another oil refinery (DAPSA), three plants that store oil and its derivatives (Petrobras, Repsol-YPF, and Petrolera Cono Sur), several plants that store chemical products (including TAGSA, Antívari, and Solvay Indupa), one plant that manufactures chemical products (Meranol), one dock for containers (Exolgan), and one thermo-electrical plant (Central Dock Sud) (Dorado 2006). According to the latest available figures, Flammable has approximately five thousand residents (Defensoría del Pueblo 2009). The population is fairly new, with 75 percent of the residents having lived in the area less than fifteen years. During the last two decades, the population increased at least fourfold. This growth was fed by shantytown removals in the city of Buenos Aires and by immigration from other provinces and nearby countries, primarily Peru, Bolivia, and Paraguay.

Flammable's soil, air, and streams are highly polluted with lead, chromium, benzene, and other chemicals (Defensoría del Pueblo 2003; Dorado 2006). An epidemiological study in 2003 compared a sample of children ages seven to eleven living in Flammable with a control population living in another poor neighborhood with similar socioeconomic characteristics but lower levels of exposure to industrial activities (JMB 2003). The study found that in both neighborhoods children are exposed to the known carcinogens chromium and benzene and to toluene. But lead distinguishes the children of Flammable from the others; in Flammable, 50 percent of the tested children had higher than normal blood levels of lead, compared with 17 percent in the control population.

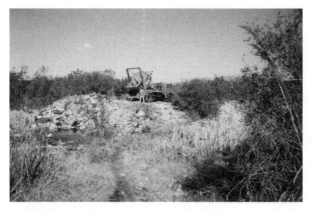

8 Dumping garbage in
   Flammable. Elemen-
   tary school photog-
   raphy workshop in
   Flammable, 2009.

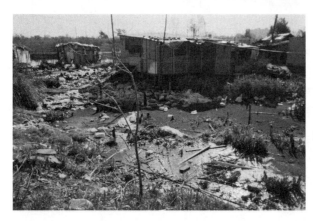

9 Living in the midst
   of garbage and
   poison. Elementary
   school photography
   workshop in
   Flammable, 2009.

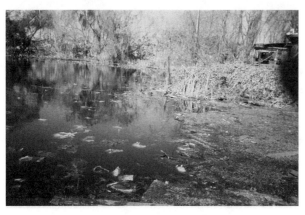

10 Backyard of a
    Flammable resident.
    Elementary school
    photography work-
    shop in Flammable,
    2009.

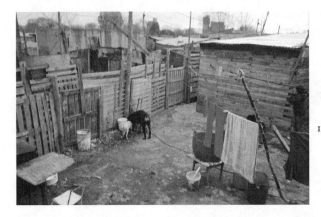

11 Flammable shanty-
town's streets.
Elementary school
photography work-
shop in Flammable,
2009.

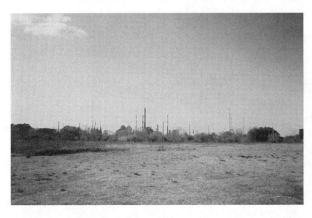

12 The Polo Petro-
químico as seen
by schoolchildren.
Elementary school
photography work-
shop in Flammable,
2009.

Described by UNEP/UNICEF as a "scourge," lead is a neurotoxin
that is easily absorbed into the bloodstream and bones. Children are
the most susceptible to the harmful effects of lead poisoning. "Exposure to excessive levels of lead," reads the UNEP/UNICEF report
titled *Childhood Lead Poisoning*, "is harmful to the health and intellectual development of millions of children and adults, in almost all
regions of the world" (1997: 1). At low levels, lead poisoning in children causes "reduction in IQ and attention span, reading and learning
disabilities, hyperactivity and behavioral problems, impaired growth
and visual and motor functioning, and hearing loss." At high levels, it

causes "anemia, brain, liver, kidney, nerve, and stomach damage, coma, convulsions, and death" (5).

Predictably, the epidemiological study conducted in Flammable found lower than average IQs among the children there along with a higher percentage of neurobehavioral problems. The study also found strong statistical associations between frequent headaches and neurological symptoms, learning problems, and hyperactivity in school. The children in Flammable reported more dermatological problems such as eye irritation, skin infections, eruptions, and allergies; more respiratory problems such as coughs and bronchospasms; more neurological problems such as hyperactivity; and more sore throats and headaches.

In June 2004 during the first months of fieldwork for *Flammable*, residents told us that their relocation was imminent. "By early 2005, nobody will be living here," we heard repeatedly. As proof of the forthcoming relocation, residents pointed to a census that municipal agents were conducting with the purpose of establishing the exact number of families living in the neighborhood. As we highlight in the book, relocation or eviction was a sort of sword of Damocles always hanging over residents' heads. In other words, the threat of removal was a defining feature of their lives.

Four and a half years later, in December 2009, we went back to the neighborhood and found that another census had been recently carried out by municipal agents. The sword of eviction or relocation was still hanging. The flyer announcing the agents' visit read as follows: "Census Objectives: To define the number of families in the neighborhood . . . To know the residents' opinions about the possibility of a relocation plan in order to propose a program that will resolve the neighborhood's needs." The government was once more raising neighbors' expectations and the local improvement association was once again calling up meetings with neighbors to discuss the possibility raised by state officials. Figure 13 shows one of these invitations.

Old-timers, however, were skeptical. They complained that "nobody comes down, nobody informs us of anything, and we keep hear-

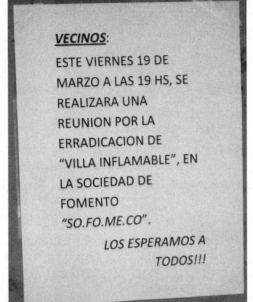

VECINOS:
ESTE VIERNES 19 DE
MARZO A LAS 19 HS, SE
REALIZARA UNA
REUNION POR LA
ERRADICACION DE
"VILLA INFLAMABLE", EN
LA SOCIEDAD DE
FOMENTO
"SO.FO.ME.CO".
       LOS ESPERAMOS A
              TODOS!!!

13 Flyer calling a meeting
to discuss eradication
in 2009. Photo by the
author.

ing the same old story"; or, "I don't believe what the government is
saying, if it were true, they would come down to the neighborhood and
give us the information." Others commented as follows:

> "I've lived here for twenty-eight years, and since the beginning they've been
> saying they were going to relocate us. I don't think so . . ." (Mario).

> "It's been thirty years since I moved here, and they always told us that we had
> to move out. But they never proposed anything specific" (Carlos).

> "Agents come around, they ask questions, but nothing ever happens" (Celina).

Disbelief notwithstanding, neighbors acknowledge that some families
—twenty-five, according to most—have been relocated. This relocation demonstrates that something might eventually happen for them.
As I described in the previous chapter, welfare benefits are eventually

granted to some, which shows to the rest that their grueling pilgrimage might pay off. Homes are being assigned and will sooner or later be allocated to a few, which also demonstrates the value of waiting. Without occasional rewards that randomly disrupt the long waiting period, the waiting would not make much sense and neither prospective welfare clients nor Flammable residents would invest in the waiting process.

One of the relocated families was that of María Soto. We met her in 2005 when she was living in a precarious wood house whose garbage-filled backyard sloped downward into a filthy swampland. María's daughter Luisa was tested for the 2003 lead study. By then, her lead levels were 18.5 micrograms per deciliter, far above what is now considered to be a nontoxic blood level of lead (10 μg/dl). At the time, María and Luisa were waiting to be allocated a unit in a housing project that the federal government was building in nearby Wilde. Those who are "the most contaminated," she believed, "will leave first." To our surprise, in early 2008 she received notification that she had been granted a unit. After months of anxious waiting ("Until I have the key in my hand, I won't celebrate!"), on May of that same year María and Luisa moved to their new home. Figures 14–16 show them packing their few belongings on top of a relative's car and happily entering their new place.

Surrounded by toxic hazards and right across from the petrochemical compound, María's old shack is still standing. One of her relatives is now living there; proving that what neighbors told us is indeed true: "For every other one who is relocated . . . more people move into the neighborhood." Neighbors also believe that who moves in and who moves out, who waits and who does not, is overdetermined by "politics": "They moved some out, but more come in . . . it's all political"; "The new homes are given to those families who are in politics."

As far as we can tell, María was not granted a home because of her political connections. Her family was identified in the epidemiological study as one of those with an urgent need for a new home. Yet we should take seriously the belief of the neighbors that it is only through politics, as something carried out "up there" by those who "never come down to the neighborhood" (*nunca bajan al barrio*), that waiting can be interrupted. Like those in the offices of the Welfare Ministry, neigh-

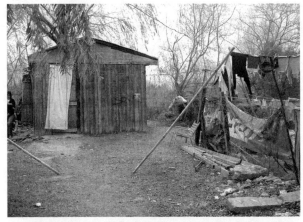

14 María's home in
Flammable. Photo
by the author.

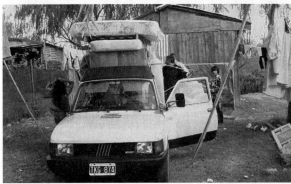

15 María leaving
Flammable.
Courtesy of Débora
Swistun.

bors are convinced that during "political times" (i.e., close to an election) "things [i.e., relocation] could get done." Politics, in this shared
understanding, is a possible accelerator that can reduce the waiting
time. For Flammable residents, encountering the state means being
caught in a "particular warp of space and time" (Secor 2007: 39). Only
political influence can afford them with the "ability to break out of
endless cycles of circulating and waiting" (39).

    In the following section, I share a series of ethnographic vignettes
that show how politics for Flammable residents invokes neither a joint
capacity to make positive changes nor a collective struggle for resources. Even less so does it invoke a process through which a specific

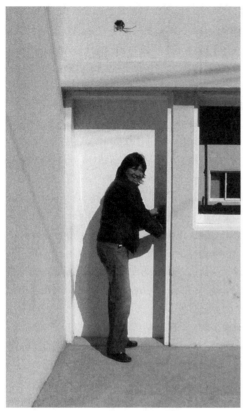

16 María entering her new home.
Courtesy of Débora Swistun.

policy is agreed upon and carried out. Politics, as the activity that can put a halt to their endless waiting, and politicians, as its main actors, loom above their lives and intermittently "come down" to the neighborhood. As an activity beyond their control, politics implies something profoundly disempowering. Thus, it is pretty much like waiting.[7]

ELSA, EUGENIO, ISABEL, AND MARGA

Rewind to June 2004. The first persons we interviewed while doing the research for our book were Eugenio, Isabel, and Marga. They were the leaders of the neighborhood's improvement association

(SOFOMECO, Sociedad de Fomento Pro Mejoramiento de la Costa) and they showed great interest in our study. The day we met them, Isabel and Marga were coming back from presenting a petition to the welfare office at the local municipality. "Municipal agents are carrying out a census," they told us, "in order to relocate people, because of all the contamination . . . but some neighbors say that it is not because of the contamination but because one of the compound companies needs to expand its operations and they bought all this land." As we examined in our study, rumors about what this or that company was about to do ran rampant. Isabel and Marga anticipated what we would repeatedly hear from many if not most residents. During our more recent visit, however, Isabel, Marga, and Eugenio told us that officials at the municipality had informed them that "eradication" of the neighborhood was going to proceed. These same officials were sending agents to conduct the census because, as Isabel told us, "they already have the authorization from the federal, state, and municipal governments to eradicate all the people from Flammable."

In June 2004, talk of relocation was constant in the neighborhood, triggered both by the census and by meetings with officials. Yet neighborhood leaders were doubtful about the form it was going to take. After all, they were property owners and not squatters like most residents of Flammable: "What are they going to do with us, property-owners? I pay taxes, I have all the proper documentation. I agree in that we have to leave because of all the contamination, but this is not a gift. I want a similar property elsewhere, or the money so that I can buy something." In this quote, Isabel reactivates a previously existing boundary between them (owners) and others (squatters).

"Did these officials tell you where they are going to relocate the neighborhood?" we asked. "No, they don't have the land yet, they don't have anything . . . it's all *chamuyo* [idle talk]. They say they are conducting a census, but . . ." said Eugenio, and Marga skeptically added: "Since I was a little kid they have been talking about eradication. This is a topic that has been going around for the longest time but never became reality . . . I think the eradication is still 'green' [not fully developed]. But, who knows? Maybe one day, all of a sudden, they come and they tell us that we have to leave. But nobody knows what's going to happen, because nobody informs us." Still, municipal officials notified them that "census and eradication" was the official policy, and they believed "something is going to happen." The reasons behind the policy were, again, the subject of incessant rumors: "Apparently, the companies made a deal with the mayor. They gave money to the mayor so that he will remove the people from here. The land is very valuable here." All the neighbors we talked to at the time conveyed their sense of uncertainty and powerlessness and a shared sentiment that the future was not in their hands. This sentiment was perhaps best captured by García, another old-time neighbor, when he said: "Now we have to wait until Shell or someone else, maybe the municipal government, expels us from here . . . . Since 1982 there have been rumors that we will be evicted."

In 2004, Eugenio and Isabel were also awaiting the decision of the courts on a lawsuit against Central Dock Sud. They were demanding 350,000 Argentine pesos (at the time, US$113,000) in compensation for the damages caused by the installation of a high-voltage-wire line that runs on top of their homes. "It's three years now since we've been in this thing . . ." Marga told us, and she continued by stating that she did not know "how the lawsuit is coming along because nobody called me yet, nobody called me . . . It's been many years now. They [the lawyers] said that they will let us know when they have news. The lawsuit takes a long time, many years." Teresa concurred with her, and in a series of long conversations pointed out the following:

Yes, we are part of a lawsuit [against Central Dock Sud] but we don't really know anything. It's been three years, and we don't know anything. The lawyer showed up at the very beginning. She told us that she would come back to inform us, but she never came back . . . . We called her several times and she is never in the office. We left messages but she never called us back. . . . [The lawsuit for indemnification] is quite difficult, but you need to hang hope on something. I don't know how much money did the lawyer ask for; she does everything, but does not inform us. We know nothing.

Finally, García expressed both his optimism and cynicism: "The lawsuit will begin to move forward this year . . . we began with it three or
four years ago. A lawyer from the company came but we didn't reach
an agreement. We signed some papers and she left. It takes a long
time. . . . I have a pending lawsuit for my pension and it's been ten years
and I still haven't seen anything."

Fast-forward to December 2009. During our last visit to the neighborhood, Isabel told us that a month ago municipal agents were conducting another census: "Census workers were asking about the number of
people living in each home, the number of rooms. They also asked
us about what we wanted for the new neighborhood. Do we want a
health center? A school? I say: I am not moving to a housing complex.
They [the new buildings where twenty-five families were relocated]
look like bird cages." Isabel and Eugenio told us that in October 2009
they had a meeting with the mayor, and he told them that "all the
people here are going to be relocated. And that the property owners
are going to be expropriated . . . but they don't really know anything.
Nobody came here to inform us!"

     This time, Eugenio and Isabel were accompanied by Elsa, the mother
of my colleague Débora Swistun. As we recounted in *Flammable*, one
day over lunch Elsa ironically portrayed herself in the distant future as
an old toothless lady with a cane, her voice trembling, happily stating
"We are about to be relocated!" Elsa and Eugenio concurred that for
every family that the government is relocating, new families are moving
in. "This is crazy," they agree, "this is not a place for a human being to
be living!" And Eugenio adds: "I don't think anybody is going to be
relocated . . . . This is all a game, they kick the ball forward, and they
don't do anything." Regarding the lawsuit, Eugenio and Isabel were less
hopeful than when we first met: "The lawyer came by last year and told
us to be patient."

     In another conversation, Elsa told me that census workers have
raised "the possibility of relocation, but there are so many versions,

so many versions . . . I really don't know." I asked her if she personally knew someone who had recently moved out of the neighborhood. Her answer resonates with what Ezpeleta's neighbors, Gladys and Angélica, believe to be EDESUR's hidden agenda regarding their protest, and it encapsulates what after all these years of waiting may be in their view the mainstream policy toward toxic suffering: "The only people I know who left are those who went up, to heaven . . . they died."

MARIANA

As I observed above, it would be very difficult to make sense of poor people's constant waiting if not for the fact that, for a few of them, waiting "pays off." Applicants at the RENAPER know that their *aguante* (endurance) will be rewarded with a DNI; and welfare clients know that the longer they wait and the more patience they show, the higher their chances of obtaining a much-needed benefit. In Flammable, the uneventful waiting is disrupted by random promises and initiatives, like the new census that was carried out in late 2009 or the lawyers' visits, and also by concrete feats such as the occasional relocation of a small group of residents. These events demonstrate to neighbors that "something is happening" and that their waiting is not totally futile.

One last story, Mariana's, illustrates well the haphazard interruption of the waiting process. Far from an isolated and idiosyncratic account, Mariana portrays "a social universe dominated by [an] absolute and unpredictable power, capable of inducing extreme anxiety by condemning its victim to very strong investment combined with great insecurity" (Bourdieu 2000: 229). It also encapsulates residents' shared understanding of their waiting as something with intimate connections to the political world, which is located far away and in which they have no say. In Mariana's account, we see power at work through the constant deferring and the routine raising of false hopes. These elements characterize the rhythm of collective life in the neighborhood, making it a site of anxious, powerless waiting.[8]

"[After the epidemiological study that identified a lead-poisoned cluster], they [the government] said that there was going to be a treatment for the kids," says Mariana, whose own son suffers from chronic asthma. "They said that there was going to be a follow-up . . . that they were going to distribute aid. . . . Nothing happened. . . . Here are lots of kids with lead in their blood, and we don't really know, because in the future that might bring you trouble, some kids might even die. . . . Officials use us . . . they make promises and they never do anything. . . . Tons of times they have said that there was going to be a relocation but nothing happened. . . . Now we are waiting for them to remove us . . . because this land has been sold. Most of the people here are going to be evicted, but who knows, they said that same thing so many times. . . . I have my doubts, I really don't know because a couple of neighbors received an eviction letter because some of this land has an owner. But I didn't receive anything. There is no property record for this particular piece of land where we live. Apparently, nobody should be living here because this is an industrial area, but nobody comes here to inform us, nobody shows up. I heard that four hundred families will be relocated . . . but there are so many families here and there is a school, a kindergarten, a church, it won't be easy for politicians to remove us. A neighbor sent a note to the politicians so that they come down and meet with us, but nobody showed up . . . Officials told us that they are too busy, that they would come later, that they would schedule an appointment . . . nothing happened. *Es un manoseo* (fumbling). . . . Nobody wants to come down, they wash their hands . . . We are waiting to see if they, the politicians, come down and give us an answer."

REASONS (NOT) TO HOPE

In July 2004, a group of residents of Flammable joined forces with physicians, psychologists, and nurses from the Hospital Interzonal de Agudos Pedro Fiorito.[9] Led by Dr. Mendoza, they brought forth a lawsuit against the federal government, the government of the province of Buenos Aires, the government of the city of Buenos Aires, and forty-four companies. Many of these companies were located inside the petrochemical compound that sits adjacent to Flammable.

The lawsuit was titled *Mendoza Beatriz Silvia and others vs. the National State and others regarding damages suffered.* These "damages" are the injuries resulting from the environmental contamination of the Matanza-Riachuelo River. Breaking with precedent, the lawsuit was received by the National Supreme Court in June 2006. The judges divided the claim in two parts: they declared there was a lack of original jurisdiction with respect to the claim aimed at redressing damage to the individual plaintiff's assets as an indirect result of aggression towards the environment, but they affirmed their competence with respect to damages to the environment.

In its first ruling, the Supreme Court determined that the object of the lawsuit was the *tutela* (protection) of the common good, and it ordered the national government, the province of Buenos Aires, the city of Buenos Aires, and the Federal Environmental Council (COFEMA) to present an integrated plan that "addresses the area's environmental situation, control over anthropogenic activities, an environmental impact study of the defendant-businesses, an environmental education program, and an environmental information program" (CSJ 2008: 2). Months later, the Supreme Court took two further actions. First, they accepted the federal ombudsman's office and a group of nongovernmental organizations, including the Fundación Ambiente y Recursos Naturales (FARN), the Centro de Estudios Legales y Sociales (CELS), and Greenpeace, as third parties in the lawsuit. Second, they included as defendants the Coordinadora Ecológica Área Metropolitana Sociedad del Estado (CEAMSE), which is the authority in charge of landfills in the metropolitan area, and fourteen municipal governments that have incidence in the Matanza-Riachuelo basin.

Over a period of three years, the Supreme Court held four public hearings in what, according to FARN director Andrés Napoli, was a "complex process that required the hard work on the part of the Supreme Court and in which the various involved parties participated actively" (FARN 2009: 88). On July 8, 2008, the Supreme Court's ruling established that the federal government, the province of Buenos Aires, and the city of Buenos Aires were responsible for the prevention and restoration of the collective environmental damage existing in the

Matanza-Riachuelo basin. The ruling mandated a series of obligatory actions to accomplish this goal, and created a broad system of control for the enforcement of the sentence, including the imposition of fines to state authorities.

In the ruling, the court understood claimants as "victims of the environmental contamination of the Matanza-Riachuelo river basin" and asserted that "the restoration from and the prevention of environmental harm requires the issuance of urgent, definitive, and effective decisions" (CSJ 2008: 1). The court, furthermore, delegated the execution of the decision to a "federal court of first instance, in order to ensure swiftness of future court decisions as well as effective judicial control over compliance" (9). The thrust of the Supreme Court's decision is found on page 10 of the sentence, where it mandates that the River Basin Authority (ACUMAR) complete a program with three simultaneous objectives: "1) Improvement of the quality of life of the river basin inhabitants; 2) the environmental restoration of all of the river basin's components (water, air, soil); 3) the prevention of reasonably foreseeable harm." The document then lists a series of specific objectives with regard to public information, industrial pollution, cleanup of landfills, cleaning of the riverbanks, expansion of the potable water network, projects for storm drainage and sewage sanitation, and an emergency health plan. On page 11, under the heading "Industrial Pollution," the sentence mandates "the public presentation, detailed and well-founded," of a project for the *reconversion and relocation of the petrochemical compound in Dock Sud* (emphasis added).

The ruling was indeed a "historic feat" (FARN 2009: 88), one that signaled that "new winds are blowing from the Judiciary in relation to environmental justice" (90). It gave some residents of Flammable and environmental activists a newfound hope for a state-led change. Whether through relocation of the neighborhood or through the relocation of the compound now ordered by the Supreme Court, new winds were indeed blowing into the neighborhood and giving residents reason to hope.

What has happened since then? A report published in December 2009 details the actions taken and not taken by state authorities on

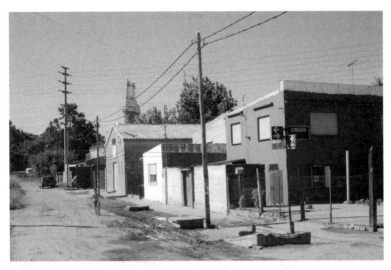

17 Flammable in 2006. Courtesy Divina Swistun.

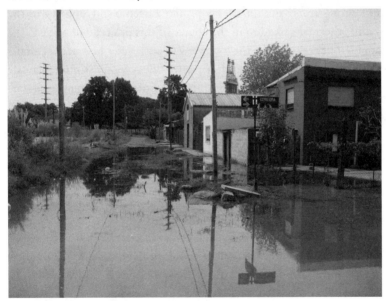

18 Flammable in 2010. Photo by the author.

each one of the Supreme Court's mandates.[10] The report concludes that no significant advances were made since the July 2008 ruling. Regarding the relocation of the petrochemical compound, which would have the most direct impact on Flammable's livability, the report expresses "concern about the authorities' delay in the implementation of the relocation and industrial reconversion of the Dock Sud petrochemical compound," and it clearly states that the orders of the Supreme Court have not been heeded (see figures 17 and 18).

Most people in Flammable and at the welfare office were interested in sharing their experiences because they wanted us and others to know what they were going through, and because they wished to express their opinions on what authorities should and should not do about their current daily problems and also on what they perceived was right and wrong or fair and unfair. People like Eugenio and Susana—or the many others we talked to in the course of this project—jumped at the opportunity afforded by the interview to both describe a state of affairs and broadcast some standard of justice. They would simultaneously talk about morality and politics, and accordingly saw us as both witnesses of their plight and advocates of their cause.

Moral standards appear profoundly intertwined with politics, and they are usually expressed by residents of Flammable in the form of moral outrage at something that was perceived as deeply manipulative ("they use us") or irresponsible ("they allow people to move into this poisoned area"). Politics also seems to permeate their understandings of the causes and possible solutions to their everyday problems. Politics, in other words, is perceived as the source of the injustice, unfairness, and arbitrariness that pervades their everyday life. Though it powerfully determines their life chances, politics is a distant and unfathomable source. It is experienced as an arena in which only other people act, and therefore as an activity in which the poor are not agents. The *periculum in mora*—danger in the delay—has in politics its main source. And, as in *Waiting for Godot*, the generalized feeling is that there is "nothing to be done" about that.

CONCLUSION

The complex relationship between subordinated groups and the state has been the subject of detailed scrutiny in both historical and ethnographic research (see, for example, Roy 1994; Bayat 1997; Wedeen 1999; Chatterjee 2006; Goldberg 2007; Wolford 2010). For the most part, this research has empirically attended to instances when this relationship has broken down—that is, when it has erupted in episodes of mass contention or explosive insurgency or when it has called for the deployment of the state's visible iron fist (Joseph and Nugent 1994; Eckstein 2001; Edelman 2001; Auyero 2003; Wood 2003; Johnston and Almeida 2006; Almeida 2008). However, there are many other forms of engagement between the state and subaltern groups, both the hidden ones embodied in the pernicious operation of clandestine kicks and the routine, ordinary ones of welfare clients and poisoned outcasts enduring long and uncertain delays.

Taken together, the fairly consistent ways in which poor people experience their waiting point to their overall mode of relating to the state: what I would call the "patient" model. To be an actual or potential welfare recipient, a shantytown dweller suffering toxic assault and (always) about to be relocated, or a legal alien awaiting an ID is to be subordinated to the will of others. The poor are, in this relationship, the subject of a constant kicking around (*peloteo*). They are pawns in the midst of the state's not-quite-evident forces, or the "playballs of a thousand chances," to recall Engels's phrase. Much like the lower-class and lower-middle-class men and women in Istanbul interviewed by Anna Secor, the subjects in this book trace their own "narratives of circulation" in the form of being "kicked around" and in following "documents, money, and influence through the offices and waiting rooms of government buildings, state ministries . . . and courts" (2007: 38). True, they are agents; but *in their interactions with the state*, their sense of agency is minimal to nonexistent. They are treated as patients, and with very few exceptions they think and feel accordingly. Readers may object by stating that I am depriving people such as Elsa or Milagros of their agency; but I would argue that the culprit is the sociopolitical order in which they are embedded. I am, on the contrary, trying to represent it in as faithful a manner as possible, based on what I have seen and heard in the field.

According to the sociologists Mario Luis Small, David Harding, and Michele Lamont (2010), "culture" has recently made a comeback in poverty research in sociology. Though I believe attention to culture was never quite absent from examinations by the social sciences of deprivation, marginality, and inequality in the Americas (see, for example, Scheper-Hughes 1992; MacLeod 1995; Bourgois 1995; Auyero 2000)—its "return" being, in fact, more the result of the parochialism of sociology in the United States and its tendency to ignore what is being done outside its national boundaries—I share Small, Harding, and Lamont's assertion that a "judicious, theoretically informed, and empirically grounded study of culture can and should be a permanent component of the poverty research agenda." Despite the renewed emphasis on poor people's "values, frames, repertoires, narratives, symbolic boundaries, cultural capital, and institutions" (8), however, their temporal experience has not yet emerged as an important research concern, much less so its *political production*.[1]

The work in this book has made abundantly clear that there is much more to waiting for state's attention than the kind of boredom and frustration that is the first-order experience of those who encounter that circumstance. Poor people's temporal experience is a key component of their "culture," and the workings and effects of domination on the dispossessed should not be ignored.[2] If what we see in a waiting room is poor people who look "passive," or "resigned," or "unwilling," whose bodies look "spilled," who seem "stick to the waiting script," (a disposition that might indeed contribute "to their own domination"), then we should never forget that their subjective state is not indigenous to them—a set of values, frames, or understandings that poor people might share because of their structural position or the neighborhoods where they live—but rather is a *political construct*. Suitably, the work in this book has also shed light on the fact that the meanings that the destitute assign to their waiting time (meanings that, as Small, Harding, and Lamont [2010] well note, both constrain and enable their actions) are an *artifact* of both state's manipulation and neoliberal policy. In the "etiology" of the temporal experience (Flaherty 2010) of those living at the bottom of the socio-symbolic order what state agents and market forces do (and do not do) matters a great deal. Thus, if we are after a "more complete understanding of the conditions that produce and sustain poverty" (Small, Harding, and Lamont 2010: 10), attention to poor people's experience of time as a *political artifact* is central. Endless delays, this book has shown, not only exacerbate the state of emergency in which the destitute live their daily lives (making the state deeply implicated in the production of human wretchedness) but also create a set of shared understandings (and its objectifications in waiting rooms, lines, always-pending lawsuits, etc.) among the oppressed concerning their own situation, their expectations, and their rights.

In other words, the "patient model" should not be understood as a demonstration of the presumably recurrent submissiveness of poor welfare clients; the various ethnographic portrayals above detected nothing of that sort (see also Edin and Lein 1997; Hays 2003; Korteweg 2006). The acquiescence dissected throughout these pages is not an essential trait of the destitute but one of those outcomes of the process of domination that Pierre Bourdieu has encouraged us to inspect closely throughout his many works (1977, 1999, 2000). My emphasis on the subordination created in the repeated encounters with the welfare office and with other state agencies should also not be read as an argument against state provision of welfare to the destitute or of other services crucial to their existence. The state is the "vexed institution" (Scott 1999) that is the ground of both poor people's domination and their possibilities of survival.

Augustín Salvia in his introduction to an illuminating collection of articles on urban marginality in Argentina notes that in a context of generalized poverty, collective survival strategies do not always result in cooperation and solidarity. In disagreement with those who describe their emancipatory potential, Salvia asserts that poor people's survival strategies involve high levels of exploitation of the labor force within the family and community and often engender competition and conflict among the destitute. These joint strategies, he argues, are increasingly subordinated to the power of the state, given its control over key welfare and economic benefits (Salvia and Molina 2007: 51). The "patient model" draws attention to one of the ways in which this subordination occurs, and to its subjective but hardly idiosyncratic effects.

Poor people's subordination to the state's mandates is created and re-created through innumerable acts of waiting, and the obverse—that domination is generated anew by making others wait—is equally true. In those recurrent encounters with street-level bureaucrats, poor people learn through endless delays and random changes that they have to comply with the requirements of an unpredictable state ("sit and wait"). In a few cases, the uncertain waiting exhausts and discourages poor people, and these end up dropping out of sight—that is, not coming back to the welfare office, ceasing the process of applying for an ID, not attending the next meeting, and so forth. For the most part, however, the unreliability and unpredictability have the paradoxical effect of *binding the destitute to the state*. With their pressing needs, they simply cannot afford to quit. The state asks the most dispossessed to "keep coming back," literally in the case of the welfare office and figuratively in the case of Flammable. Those about to be evicted, those who cannot feed their children, and those living in the midst of a sickening toxic soup are not able to decline this command. They comply ("if you want the benefit, you have to keep coming"), thereby effectively strapping themselves to the very institution that is reducing or depriving them of their already meager benefits while at the same time routinely disempowering them.

State agents do not place much emphasis on the "customs, habits, ways of acting and thinking" (Foucault 2000: 209) of those in need. The "rehabilitative function" of welfare in the United States (Goldberg 2007: 3; see also Gilliom 2001; Hays 2003) has historically placed much emphasis on controlling the most minute aspects of poor people's behaviors—governing their bodies and souls—and on molding the "habits, behavior, or dispositions" of the poor. In my fieldwork, however, I did not see much attention to these aspects. Rather, the interactions with the state described under the "patient model" introduce "economy and order" (i.e., government, in Foucault's sense) through the manipulation of poor people's time. It is through this practice, through this "governing technique" (Foucault 1979: 198), that the state creates docility among the poor. The "patient model" could thus be seen as a particular historically situated illustration of the productive nature of power. Interpreted in this light, the "mundane statements [made] by minor administrators" (Rabinow 1984: 15) acquire a more relevant and more consequential sociopolitical significance. Although much less spectacular than troops, thugs, and jails, the seemingly unimportant assertions and commands uttered by low-ranking street-level bureaucrats and the beliefs of those subjected to their commands should be understood as indicators of the workings of power. The justifications and injunctions of state officials, the stories of resignation and frustration of the subordinated, the "uneventful" encounters at the waiting room, and the ordinary visit of a census worker are far from trivial. They embody, in fact, the *everyday reconstruction of political domination*. In these diverse settings, waiting appears to be "in the order of things"—as something normal, expected, inevitable. Poor people's ways of thinking and feeling about it seem to be arranged in accordance with the very relational structures of domination between the destitute and the state. Waiting should thus be thought of as a script that is invested with the objectivity of the common sense, and the dispossessed know it all too well. This script, I hope my analysis has shown, is both a product of everyday domination (but not, to repeat, an essential trait of the poor) and the producer of daily submission.

In this book I have described in micro-sociological detail the workings of a not-quite-visible form of state power. I have provided diverse ethnographic accounts of *one* type of relationship between the urban poor and the state, which certainly is not the only mode of interaction. My research in Argentina (Auyero 2000, 2003, 2007) and that of others in other parts of the world (Lazar 2008; Shefner 2008; Kerkvliet 2005; Holzner 2004; Goldstein 2003; Gay 1994) have uncovered a diversity of ways in which the destitute engage with the state, from patronage to civic participation to contentious collective action. For both political and scholarly reasons, patiently and silently waiting for the state to deliver on its promises has not received the same empirical and theoretical attention.

After analytically isolating and scrutinizing this particular temporal experience as a form of poor people's regulation, much work lies ahead. A few avenues for future research would include, as a starting point, an examination of other specific social universes in which waiting (or, more generally, the management of poor people's temporal experience by the dominant) takes a prominent place, and then compare to the ones I have analyzed in this book. Public hospitals, for example, would be an obvious place for such an inquiry, and other arenas would include marginalized communities awaiting infrastructural improvements, relocation, or eviction. Squatter settlements expecting "regularization" of their land tenure and slum dwellers anticipating the "urbanization" of their *villas miseria* would also be appealing case studies. How is the temporal experience of the powerless customized in such arenas? Through what specific mechanisms do they become ensnared in the state's temporal demands? What kind of reciprocal obligations, both material and symbolic, are established in the process? What, if any, are the strategies devised and implemented by the dispossessed to resist or otherwise cope with the manipulation exerted by the powerful? If, as Mustafa Emirbayer and Ann Mische note, the full complexity of the agentic dimension of social action can only be captured if "it is analytically situated in *the flow of time*" (1998: 963; my emphasis), then the temporal experience of the destitute is an inescapable dimension of a better understanding of their "agency" (or lack thereof).

The division of labor of the domestication of the poor is distributed among market and state forces. In the daily lives of the dispossessed, as I noted earlier, visible fists, clandestine kicks, and invisible tentacles frequently meet and mesh. It would be worthwhile for future research to empirically dissect variations in the material and symbolic importance of fists, kicks, and tentacles, the spaces in which they act, and the categories and relational settings they affect. For example: Are fists and kicks more active in some urban spaces (for example, in shanty-towns and squatter settlements) than in others (working-class neighborhoods)? Do tentacles gravitate toward certain categories of people (for example, women and the elderly) more than others (men and the young)? Do certain relationships (for example, patronage networks) protect the poor against fists and kicks but channel them into the tentacles' power?

From the work of Loïc Wacquant (2009) and Alice Goffman (2009) we know that mass incarceration (the state's visible fist) is having devastating effects in the African American ghetto in the contemporary United States (see also Mauer and Chesney-Lind 2002). We also know, from the work of Megan Comfort (2008) for example, that the prison regulates poor people's daily lives in visible and not so visible ways. The impact of hyper prisonization cannot be measured exclusively in numerical form. We need, both Comfort and Goffman tell us, to examine the on-the-ground effects that this mode of domination is having in poor communities. On the one hand, the generalized fear, the mutual suspicion, the feeling of being constantly "on the run" (Goffman 2009) pervades the lives of marginalized youngsters as they sometimes evade and other times resist the state's "punishment of the poor" (Wacquant 2009). On the other hand, the prison "socializes" not only those who are behind bars but also their partners, relatives, and loved ones who regularly come in contact with it and end up "doing time together" (Comfort 2008). In Argentina, the prison is also becoming a constant presence in the daily life of the poor. When, fifteen years ago, I began my first long-term ethnography that resulted in *Poor People's Politics* (2000), the prison was not a steady presence. Today, however, it is quite common to talk with residents of poor neighborhoods whose sons, daughters, brothers, sisters, fathers, partners, mothers, or relatives are "doing time."[3] Given the recent explosive growth of incarceration in Argentina (expansion that, as mentioned in chapter 2, affects poor people in disproportionate ways), we should ask, along with Wacquant, Goffman, and Comfort, about the specific impact of prisonization in the everyday life of dwellers of shantytowns, slums, squatter settlements, and other poor barrios.

By their very nature, clandestine kicks are very difficult to study. In Argentina and elsewhere in the Americas, investigative reporters and social scientists have documented the ways in which power holders have relied on their illicit links with party members and other types of grassroots activists to conduct the "dirty work" of politics.[4] This dirty work includes everything from the intimidation or public shaming of election opponents (known in the local parlance as *contrapiquete*) to the use of shock troops in the eradication of illegal settlements. It also includes the inciting and directing of large-scale violence such as in the food riots of December 2001 (Auyero 2007), the arson of Villa Cartón described in chapter 3, and the "land invasions" that every now and then take place in contemporary Buenos Aires.[5] In previous work (Auyero 2007), I highlight the key role played by violence specialists—with their good, but not quite visible, connections to established power-holders—in the generation of episodes of collective violence. And my brief review of the current relevance of clandestine kicks in the regulation of poor people's lives presented in chapter 2 convinced me that much more empirical work lies ahead of us because, sadly, this form of political control shows no signs of fading in the near future. We should pay closer attention to the often (in)visible relationships between state officials, party operatives, and perpetrators of violence and the ways in which these relations are activated and deployed in the management of poor people's behavior. By their very nature, these relationships are obscure, and political necessities often dictate their active obscurement so that it is incumbent on those of us who study popular politics to, in the words of a grassroots leader I interviewed in previous research (2007), learn how to "listen (and to look) carefully." It is ethnographic research that is equipped to listen and look assiduously, and it is ethnographic research that can excavate *in vivo* the political dynamics that both create and sustain the need for such (in)visible connections and (in)visible acts (Auyero and Mahler 2011). But we should not dig alone. It is my firm belief that in identifying, describing, and explaining the specific set of practices and relationships that define what I call "clandestine kicks" we should enlist the help of other observers and analysts outside the limited (and limiting) boundaries of academia. As illustrated in chapter 2, these individuals should include most notably investigative reporters and state prosecutors who can often—thanks to their own set of often (in)visible connections—guide us into this still relatively unknown and understudied realm of state action, as long as we follow their path with the proper epistemological vigilance.

Interactions with the state have their one-way streets, their no-entry signs, their things to say and not to say and things to do and to avoid doing, their obligations and penalties. These could be literal or figurative, as we have seen throughout the book. Taken together, they constitute an order—call it the order of political domination—that with few exceptions appears to be firmly established. Stemming from two "recurrent surprises," to resort to an intentionally oxymoronic expression, which are the stability of the political order and the persistency of poor people's waiting, the analysis presented in this book has attempted to show that both are, in fact, deeply intertwined in the daily experience of the most destitute.

On March 2010, I visited the two elementary schools where my research collaborator Flavia Bellomi works as a teacher (see chapter 2).
The two schools are located fifteen blocks apart in the area known as
Cuartel Noveno, and one of them is adjacent to "El campito"—one of
the most recent squatter settlements in the southern part of the Conurbano Bonaerense. The area is known for its widespread poverty and
unemployment, its dreadful living conditions, and its high levels of
interpersonal violence.

Both schools are located a short twenty-minute bus ride from the
center of Lomas de Zamora, where Flavia lives with her family and
where I stay while in Argentina. The short distance belies the deep
contrast between the middle-class life of the town's center and the
utter destitution of its periphery.

Flavia and I arrive at the first school at 7:30 AM, and dozens of
children are already lining up outside. After the morning pledge, we
and her fifteen second graders (on a typical day half of her class is
absent) move into her shabby classroom. Only a laminated poster with
the alphabet and a few pictures of the nation's founding fathers deco-
rate the bare, badly painted walls. All the students have their breakfast
at school, so after the ten minutes in the classroom that students use to
get themselves ready for the day we all head to the cafeteria. It's 9:10
AM when Flavia and her students are back in the classroom. The students leave school at 12:15 PM, right after lunch. Breakfast, lunch, and
two recesses leave only one hundred minutes of effective class time per
day. During the past year, classes have been canceled because of teach-

ers' and janitors' strikes, flooding in the neighborhood, and major problems in the school building such as lack of water and the breakdown of the purifying plant. As a result, students at both schools have had classes an average of three days per week.

"Today is March 19, 2010," Flavia writes on the blackboard in both capital letters and cursive. She will later tell me during the break that "it's really, really hard for them to copy this in their notebooks." I notice that it is an especially difficult task for eight-year-old Mariana. She is sitting in the first row and she walks to the blackboard four times over the course of the ten minutes it takes her to complete a seemingly easy task. Mariana, I quickly realize, needs eyeglasses. I sit close to her and lend her mine. "Everything looks gigantic!" she says with a big smile. Flavia tells me that she has sent a few notes to Mariana's parents letting them know that she might need to see an eye doctor. Both of Mariana's parents are recent migrants from Bolivia and they manufacture clothes in a nearby sweatshop. "They told me they don't have money to pay for a doctor's visit and even less for a pair of glasses," Flavia tells me, "and then they began to cry. They were so ashamed." Flavia told them about the free optometrist in the public hospital in the center of town, and she adds that the school's social worker can help them make an appointment.

Three months later, Mariana does not yet have an appointment at the public hospital. The old social worker left the school in March and the new one is demanding that Flavia "put everything [about Mariana] in writing." Every case, Flavia writes in her fieldnote diary in late May 2010, "needs to begin anew. There's a file with all the details of Mariana's history but the social worker tells me that I need to start a new file."

Flavia's impotence and frustration at what she calls "state abandonment," expressed in the school's crumbling building, the lack of school supplies, and the inferior education the school provides to its destitute students, filters through the pages of a letter she sent me as I was finishing this admittedly pessimistic book. "In the meantime," she writes, "Mariana is still sitting in the first row, as you saw her, waiting."

The ethnographic fieldwork for this project was composed of four con-
tinuous months of observations and informal interviews on the outside of the Registro Nacional de las Personas (RENAPER) and twelve
months, divided in two periods of six months, of observations and both
formal and informal interviews in the waiting area of the welfare office.
Fieldwork was conducted during 2008 and 2009. At the RENAPER we
conducted only ten informal interviews, but one of the research assistants went through the entire ID application process along with other
foreign residents. At the welfare office we conducted eighty-nine interviews lasting between thirty minutes and two hours with welfare applicants and recipients, and ten interviews with social workers and
officials who work at the welfare ministry. The revisit to Flammable included six interviews with residents, the recoding of fieldnotes
and interviews conducted for a previous project (Auyero and Swistun
2009), and conversations with current residents conducted by the author. Four research assistants collaborated in this project, Agustín Burbano de Lara, Nadia Finck, Shila Vilker, and Regina Ricco. Agustín
conducted observations and interviews at the RENAPER and at the
welfare office. Nadia and Shila conducted observations and interviews
only at the welfare office. Shila also conducted interviews with welfare
officials. Regina carried out the interviews in Flammable.

Fieldwork at the RENAPER and at the welfare office began with one
and a half months of unobtrusive observation. After we familiarized
ourselves with the routines—or the lack thereof—in the waiting lines,
we began to chat with those who, for lack of a better term, we called *los*

esperantes. Toward the end of the four months of fieldwork at the RENAPER, we carried out ten informal interviews that confirmed what we observed during the previous months of both first unobtrusive and then participant observation.

The initial six weeks of nonparticipant observation at the welfare office were followed by five months of focused observations and indepth interviews, during which we visited the sites two or three times per week. The initial objective of the nonparticipant observation at both sites was to register, as best as we could, what happened when people were waiting. We concentrated on the following very general questions: What do los esperantes do (sleep, eat, read, chat, complain, etc.)? Are they alone or in groups? How do they talk about what is going on? What do they say about officials and about the others who are waiting with them? If they are with children, how do they interact with them? What do children do while their parents wait?

Informal interviews at the RENAPER were shorter than at the welfare office, and the main objective was to reconstruct the application process from the point of view of the applicant by focusing on access to information, requirements, and the general experience of waiting on the sidewalks of the office. Interviews at the welfare office typically began with a general inquiry about the welfare clients' reasons to be applying for a specific benefit. This served to reconstruct the clients' trajectory into the world of welfare. I then focused on the following nine dimensions: (1) general evaluations of the working of the welfare office, such as the things attendants think are working well and the things they believe should be improved; (2) perceptions regarding requirements to access welfare and information about paydays; (3) reasons they have been given to explain lack of payments or cancellation of a program; (4) times they have been asked to come back for the same claim and reasons they have been given for such a request; (5) comparison between the time they have to wait at the office with their "waiting times" at other public institutions (we let them come up with a comparison); (6) views of others who are waiting alongside them; (7) views of the welfare agents; (8) whether they come alone or in groups; and (9) ways of finding out about the particular program they are trying to access. We also asked them about their previous visits to the office and their reasons for coming, and about whether or not, at the time of the interview, they knew if or when they were going to receive the benefit or payment. This latter question served as a rough indicator of the uncertainty regarding the workings of each program. We also registered basic demographic indicators: age, citizenship, time of residence in the country, and place of residence. Together, these observations and interviews allowed us to reconstruct as completely as possible the shared experience of waiting.

Interviews with state agents focused on the following eight general themes: (1) types of subsidies distributed by their office; (2) procedures and requirements to obtain them; (3) typical problems that applicants and beneficiaries have (housing, food, medical assistance, etc.); (4) ways of distributing information about existing welfare programs; (5) the most important changes in welfare allocation since the last administration; (6) perceptions regarding the increase in evictions and their effects in the programs they work for; (7) knowledge about recipients' extended delays and their understanding of the reason behind long waiting periods; and (8) their knowledge and evaluations about clients' perceptions of the programs and the recurrent "reprogramming" of benefits. Since most of them are university-trained professionals, many took a great interest in our focus on the uncertainty and arbitrariness of waiting. Further, because they knew Shila Vilker personally or were somewhat acquainted with her, the interviews often allowed for their general reflection on the reasons behind the extended delays suffered by los esperantes.

In Flammable, interviews focused on the following four dimensions: (1) knowledge and evaluations about recent official announcements regarding relocation; (2) knowledge and evaluations about court resolutions; (3) knowledge and evaluations about recent and future relocations of neighbors and of themselves; and (4) general views about contamination and state initiatives to clean up the area or to treat the lead-poisoned youngsters living in the area. I also went back to the interviews and fieldnotes produced in the course of the original study and recoded them, focusing most of my attention on all the instances in which residents were awaiting some decision.

Waiting is an intricate focus of study because to a great extent it is "uneventful." At the early stages of the fieldwork, we went through many periods in which we thought that no sociologically interesting object could be constructed out of this "dead time." After repeated observations, and detailed and extensive fieldnotes, we began to unearth certain objective and subjective patterns (the changing procedures, the widespread uncertainty, etc.) that became the focus of our sustained attention. But this was not a purely inductive process. As I described in the introduction, we began our fieldwork with certain theoretical ideas in mind regarding the relationship between time and power, the links between subordination and waiting, and the hidden ways in which uncertainty is politically produced and at the same time is a reproducer of political domination. These half-formed theoretical ideas allowed us to better see what was going on in the field. To repeat what I stated in the introduction and in many sociological texts, without theory we would have been blind and lost (and, given the dullness of the waiting areas, terribly bored). Slowly and laboriously we improved our view and at the same time enriched our understanding of those theoretical connections; indeed, empirical and theoretical work comprises one mutually reinforcing endeavor.

NOTES

INTRODUCTION

1 In one of the many versions of the Greek myth, early-in-life Tiresias surprises Athena while she is taking a bath. In punishment for having seen his daughter naked, Zeus blinds young Tiresias but comforts him with the gift of seercraft.

2 I borrow the term "tempography" from Eviatar Zerubavel (1979).

3 I wish to thank Ian Roxborough for making me aware of this important point about my own work.

TWO. URBAN RELEGATION

1 All these entail, to paraphrase Peck and Tickell (2002: 384), the "active destruction and discreditation" of the import substitution industrialization model of economic growth and its related Keynesian welfarist-populist institutions.

2 Shantytowns are the main form of informal settlement in the city of Buenos Aires, while "squatter settlements" predominate in the Conurbano Bonaerense. On the difference between these two urban informal forms, see Cravino et al. 2008.

3 For diverse descriptions of living conditions in shantytowns, see Alarcón 2003; Auyero 2000; Auyero and Swistun 2009; and Epele 2010.

4 Given the lack of reliable official data, considerable polemics revolve around existing figures (*La Nación*, February 3, 2009; *Página12*, March 21, 2009).

5 "Class Divide Hardens for Argentina's Growing Poor," *Christian Science Monitor*, January 7, 2008.

6 This name is a pseudonym.

7 A decade ago, authors such as Kees Koonings (2001) and Roberto Briceño-León (1999) argued that a new kind of violence was emerging in Latin America. This violence was "increasingly available to a variety of social actors

and [it was] no longer a resource of elites or security forces" (Koonings 2001: 403). This new violence was, according to this strand of scholarship, quite varied; it included "everyday criminal and street violence, riots, social cleansing, private account selling, police arbitrariness, paramilitary activities, post-Cold War guerrillas, etc." (403). How "new" this violence was (and still is) has been the subject of much debate among academics. As Polly Wilding asserts: "Whether a perceived shift in actors and motives (from predominantly political to predominantly criminal) reflects a significant shift in the lived experiences of violence and insecurity is debatable. Arguably, actors have mutated but not changed; in some instances uniformed police officers are less likely to be involved in overt violence, but the same individuals may be functioning under the remit of death squads or militia groups. In any case, state violence against particular social groups, including poor, marginalized communities, as a form or result of exclusion and oppression, is an enduring, rather than new, aspect of modern society" (2010: 725).

Although the discussion is important for those attempting to diagnose the course and form of diverse types of violence in the region as a whole (Pearce 2010), the "newness" of violence is beyond dispute for those residing in territories of relegation in urban Buenos Aires.

8 Following Peck and Tickell, we could characterize these three forms of regulation as constitutive parts of the "roll-out" phase of neoliberalism. As they assert, in this new guise neoliberalism "is increasingly associated with the political foregrounding of new modes of 'social' and penal policy-making, concerned specifically with the aggressive reregulation, disciplining, and containment of those marginalized or dispossessed by the [previous] neoliberalization" (2002: 389).

9 As the journalist and human rights activist Horacio Verbitsky (2010) puts it: "There is no obvious relationship between the number of people in prison and crime rates. The former is related to political decisions and these in turn respond to electoral strategies" (2010: 10).

10 Compare these figures with the education level of the general population of the province of Buenos Aires: 3 percent without instruction, 12 percent with incomplete elementary education, 31 percent with complete elementary education, 21 percent with incomplete high school, and 16 percent with finished high school (Instituto Nacional de Estadísticas y Censos [INDEC], www.indec.gov.ar).

11 See also the annual report of the Comisión Provincial por la Memoria (2010).

12 From Cristian Alarcón, "El Barrio Fuerte," *Revista C*, November 2008; my translation.

13 On the growth of evictions in the city of Buenos Aires, see Centre on Housing Rights and Evictions 2007.

14 From "Cuando el desalojo porteño es express," *Página12*, January 15, 2010.

15 From Lucía Alvarez, "Desalojados"; my translation.

16 This encouragement to apply for a housing subsidy in the midst of an eviction could also be seen as an example of what Erving Goffman famously called "cooling out the mark." As Goffman writes, "In the argot of the criminal world the term 'mark' refers to any individual who is a victim or prospective victim of certain forms of planned illegal exploitation. The mark is the sucker—the person who is taken in [and who then needs to be cooled out, that is, he or she is] given instruction in the philosophy of taking a loss [and persuaded to] accept the inevitable and quietly go home" (1952: 451). Goffman extends the term and applies it to other persons who, finding themselves in difficult situations, are "made to accept the great injury that has been done to their image of themselves, regroup their defenses, and carry on without raising a squawk" (452). The housing subsidy could be understood as the instrument used by state officials in this process of cooling out the evicted.

THREE. POOR PEOPLE'S WAITING

1 Quotes in this paragraph come from three main sources, the newspapers *Clarín*, *Página12*, and *La Nación*.

2 Personal interview with the state prosecutor Mónica Cuñarro.

3 This fact was confirmed by virtually everyone I interviewed about this case, and it further substantiates the central role played by clandestine connections in the makings of collective violence, examined under the term "gray zone of state power" (Auyero 2007).

4 Personal interview with a former city official.

5 Personal interview with the state prosecutor.

6 Milagros's story is a composite created on the basis of many stories heard in the waiting line outside the RENAPER and at the welfare office waiting area.

7 All fieldnotes at the RENAPER were taken during 2008.

FOUR. THE WELFARE OFFICE

1 For electoral results in the city of Buenos Aires, see Ministerio del Interior, http://www.mininterior.gov.ar/. For monthly distribution of benefits in the city of Buenos Aires, see City of Buenos Aires, http://www.buenosaires .gov.ar/.

2 Interestingly enough, AFDC applicants in the United States share a similar perception of the welfare agency. "After offering several analogies to illustrate the status she felt during the waiting stage, Alissa settled on the metaphor, "They're the cowboys, and you are the cow. . . . You feel like cattle or

something being prodded. . . . These people (referring to cowboy bureaucrats) are like 'I'm helping you. This is something for you. So just be quiet
and follow your line'" (Soss 1999: 61).

3 See Gorban 2009 for an example of active problem-solving among scavengers.

4 For an example of "resistant patients," see Mulcahy, Parry, and Glover 2010.

5 See, for example, Ministerio de Desarrollo Social, "Guía de servicios sociales
   2009," http://estatico.buenosaires.gov.ar/areas/des_social/fortal_soc_civil/
   guia_version_web.pdf.

6 See "Monitoreo del programa cuidadanía porteña," http://estatico2.buenos
   aires.gov.ar/areas/des_social/evaluacion_programas/informes_condiciones
   _vida/Informe_Monitoreo_Noviembre_2009.pdf.

7 All quotes come from descriptions used in the "Guía de servicios sociales
   2009," published by the Ministerio de Desarrollo Social (cited above).

8 Or as Ann Orloff puts it: "Social policy has symbolic significance in uphold-
   ing or undermining the gender order. . . . The state is critical to gender
   relations; ideological and cultural assumptions institutionalized in state programs shape gender and other social relations" (1999: 323).

FIVE. FLAMMABLE REVISITED

1 María Eugenia Cerutti and Silvina Heguy, *132.000 volts: El caso Ezpeleta*, 77.

2 Agustín Burbano de Lara conducted the interviews with Gladys and Angélica at Gladys's home in July 2010.

3 A powerful photographic report of this collective suffering can be found
   in the award-winning book by Cerutti and Heguy, *132.000 volts: El caso
   Ezpeleta* (2006).

4 A *recurso de amparo* is an injunction or mandamus to protect constitutional
   rights.

5 For a recent chronicle on the state of the river and its neighbors, see Hoshaw
   2008.

6 Between June and September 2009, Divina Swistun, a professional pho-
   tographer, taught a group of elementary schoolchildren the basics of photography. Their final project was to take twenty-four pictures on the things
   they like about their neighborhood and the things they dislike. See Auyero
   and Swistun 2009 for the results of the first photographic exercise with a
   different group of students from the same elementary school.

7 In *Routine Politics and Collective Violence in Argentina* (2007) I make a
   similar argument about the meaning of politics among the main actors in the
   2001 food riots.

8 On the statistical association between an individual's sense of powerlessness

(or belief in external control) and low socioeconomic status, see Mirowsky and Ross 1983.

9 The account that follows was reconstructed on the basis of newspaper accounts (from *Clarín* and *Página12*), reports published by the Fundación Ambiente y Recursos Naturales (FARN) and the Centro de Información Judicial (CIJ) in their Web sites, and the Supreme Court sentence (available in English at www.farn.org.ar).

10 The report was published jointly by the Cuerpo colegiado para la participación ciudadana en la ejecución de la sentencia de la corte suprema de justicia de la nación en la causa Matanza Riachuelo, the group of NGOs recognized as third parties in the original lawsuit, who are in charge of monitoring the progress in the fulfillment of the objectives mandated by the Supreme Court. See FARN 2009.

CONCLUSION

1 An important exception to this general lack of attention can be seen in Young 2004.

2 I should add, in passing, that if anything should be "brought back into" poverty research, it is a concern with power and domination that, as Loïc Wacquant (2002) rightly points out, has almost disappeared from most social science accounts of poor people's lives.

3 As I write this I am in the process of beginning a new research project on daily violence and the effects of incarceration in Cuartel Noveno, a high-poverty area in the former industrial belt of Buenos Aires. As I stated in chapter 2, my research collaborator Flavia Bellomi, teaches in two elementary schools in the area. A third of her class members (twenty-five students) have a close relative behind bars. Although I do not have similar data that would allow for a comparison with 1995 (the time of my first fieldwork in the area), my own ethnographic observations and interviews at the time did not detect a pressing concern with imprisonment (or the actual absence of family members due to incarceration).

4 For a review of the literature, see Auyero 2007.

5 This is so much the case that it would not be farfetched to argue that Argentine politicos (past and present officials of mainstream political parties with all their democratic credentials in order) conceive of poor people's violence (or the threat thereof) as a specific weapon with which to advance their position(s) in the political field. Collective violence, and what is more, the possibility thereof, is a form of political capital that circulates within the field of official politics. The more physical damage one can (potentially) create, the more other political actors must take one into account.

WORKS CITED

Actis, Munú, Cristina Aldini, Liliana Gardella, Miriam Lewin, and Elisa Tokar. 2006. *Ese Infierno: Conversaciones de cinco mujeres sobrevivients de la ESMA*. Buenos Aires: Altamira.

Alarcón, Cristian. 2003. *Cuando me muera quiero que me toquen cumbia: Vidas de pibes chorros*. Buenos Aires: Norma.

———. 2008. "El Barrio Fuerte," *Revista C*, November, 15–19.

———. 2009. *Si me querés quereme transa*. Buenos Aires: Norma.

Alford, Robert, and Andras Szanto. 1996. "Orpheus Wounded: The Experience of Pain in the Professional Worlds of the Piano." *Theory and Society* 25 (1): 1–44.

Almeida, Paul. 2008. *Waves of Protest: Popular Struggle in El Salvador, 1925–2005*. Minneapolis: University of Minnesota Press.

Altimir, Oscar, Luis Beccaria, and Martín Gonzales Rozada. 2002. "Income Distribution in Argentina, 1974–2002." *Cepal Review* 78 (December): 1–32.

Alvarez, Lucía. 2009. "Desalojados." *Las Aguilas Humanas* blog, September 8. http://aguilashumanas.blogspot.com.

Arango, Arturo. 1995. *Lista de Espera*. Havana: Ediciones Unión.

Arditti, Rita. 1999. *Searching for Life: The Grandmothers of the Plaza de Mayo and the Disappeared Children of Argentina*. Berkeley: University of California Press.

Arias, Desmond. 2006. *Drugs and Democracy in Rio de Janeiro*. Chapel Hill: University of North Carolina Press.

Arondskin, Ricardo. 2001. *Más Cerca o Más Lejos del Desarrollo? Transformaciones Económicas en los 90*. Buenos Aires: Centro Rojas.

Auyero, Javier. 1999. "This Is Like the Bronx, Isn't It? Lived Experiences of Marginality in an Argentine Slum." *International Journal of Urban and Regional Research* 23: 45–69.

——. 2000. *Poor People's Politics*. Durham: Duke University Press.

——. 2003. *Contentious Lives: Two Argentine Women, Two Protests, and the Quest for Recognition*. Durham: Duke University Press.

——. 2007. *Routine Politics and Collective Violence in Argentina: The Gray Zone of State Power*. Cambridge: Cambridge University Press.

——. 2008. "The Political Ethnographer's *Compagnon*." Social Science Research Council website, Tributes to Charles Tilly. http://essays.ssrc.org.

Auyero, Javier, and Lauren Joseph. 2008. "Politics under the Ethnographic Microscope." *Politics under the Microscope: Readings in Political Ethnography*, edited by Lauren Joseph, Javier Auyero, and Matthew Mahler, 1–18. New York: Springer.

Auyero, Javier, Pablo Lapegna, and Fernanda Page. 2009. "Patronage Politics and Contentious Collective Action: A Recursive Relationship." *Latin American Politics and Society* 51 (3): 1–31.

Auyero, Javier, and Matthew Mahler. 2011. "Invisible Acts, Invisible Connections." *Meanings of Violence in Contemporary Latin America*, edited by Gabriela Polit Dueñas and María Helena Rueda, 197–234. New York: Palgrave.

Auyero, Javier, and Débora Swistun. 2009. *Flammable: Environmental Suffering in an Argentine Shantytown*. New York: Oxford University Press.

Bachelard, Gaston. 2006 [1938]. *Formation of the Scientific Mind*. Manchester: Clinamen Press.

Baiocchi, Gianpaolo. 2005. *Militants and Citizens: The Politics of Participatory Democracy in Porto Alegre*. Stanford: Stanford University Press.

Bandura, Albert. 1982. "Self-Efficacy Mechanism in Human Agency." *American Psychologist* 37 (2): 122–47.

——. 1998. "Personal and Collective Efficacy in Human Adaptation and Change." *Advances in Psychological Science: Vol. 1. Personal, Social, and Cultural Aspects*, edited by J. G. Adair, D. Belanger, and K. L. Dion, 51–71. Hove, U.K.: Psychology Press.

Bayat, Asef. 1997. *Street Politics*. New York: Columbia University Press.

Becker, Howard. 1958. "Problems of Inference and Proof in Participant Observation." *American Sociological Review* 23 (6): 652–60.

Beckett, Samuel. 1952. *En attendant Godot*. Paris: Les Éditions de Minuit.

Bianchi, Susana, and Norma Sanchis. 1988. *El partido peronista femenino*. Buenos Aires: CEAL.

Bloom, Harold, ed. 1987. *Samuel Beckett's Waiting for Godot*. New York: Chelsea House Publishers.

Borges, Jorge Luis. 1999. "Funes, His Memory." *Collected Fictions*, 131–37. New York: Penguin.

Bourdieu, Pierre. 1977. *Outline of the Theory of Practice*. Cambridge: Cambridge University Press.

———. 1990. *The Logic of Practice*. California: Stanford University Press.

———. 1991. *Language and Symbolic Power*. Cambridge: Harvard University Press.

———. 1998. *Practical Reason*. Stanford: Stanford University Press.

———. 1999. *Acts of Resistance*. New York: New Press.

———. 2000. *Pascalian Meditations*. Stanford: Stanford University Press.

———. 2001. *Masculine Domination*. Stanford: Stanford University Press.

Bourdieu, Pierre, and Loïc Wacquant. 1992. *Introduction to Reflexive Sociology*. Chicago: University of Chicago Press.

Bourgois, Philippe. 2001. "The Power of Violence in War and Peace." *Ethnography* 2 (1): 5–34.

———. 2003 [1995]. *In Search of Respect: Selling Crack in El Barrio*. Cambridge: Cambridge University Press.

Bourgois, Phillipe, and Jeffrey Schonberg. 2009. *Righteous Dopefiend*. Berkeley: University of California Press.

Briceño-León, Roberto. 1999. "Violence and the Right to Kill: Public Perceptions from Latin America." Unpublished manuscript, available at http://lanic.utexas.edu/project/etext/violence/memoria/session_1.html.

Brinks, Daniel. 2008a. "Inequality, Institutions, and the Rule of Law: The Social and Institutional Bases of Rights." Working paper 351. Helen Kellogg Institute. University of Notre Dame.

———. 2008b. *The Judicial Response to Police Violence in Latin America: Inequality and the Rule of Law*. New York: Cambridge University Press.

Brown, Phil, and Edwin Mikkelsen. 1990. *No Safe Place. Toxic Waste, Leukemia, and Community Action*. Berkeley: University of California Press.

Brubaker, Roger, and Frederick Cooper. 2000. "Beyond 'Identity.'" *Theory and Society* 29: 1–47.

Burawoy, Michael. 1982. *Manufacturing Consent*. Chicago: University of Chicago Press.

———. 2009. *The Extended Case Method*. Berkeley: University of California Press.

Burawoy, Michael, Alice Burton, Ann Arnett Ferguson, and Kathryn J. Fox. 1991. *Ethnography Unbound: Power and Resistance in the Modern Metropolis*. Berkeley: University of California Press.

Catenazzi, Andrea, and Juan D. Lombardo. 2003. *La cuestión urbana en los noventa en la región metropolitana de Buenos Aires*. Buenos Aires: Universidad Nacional de General Sarmiento, Instituto del Conurbano.

Centre on Housing Rights and Evictions (COHRE). 2007. "Informe sobre Argentina." http://www.cohre.org/.

Centro de Estudios Legales y Sociales (CELS). 2003. "Protesta social." http://www.cels.org.ar/.

———. 2009. *Derechos humanos en Argentina: Informe 2009*. Buenos Aires: Siglo XXI.

———. 2010. "Denuncia incumplimiento, propone medidas, solicita audiencia pública." http://www.cels.org.ar/.

Cerutti, María Eugenia, and Silvina Heguy. 2006. *132.000 volts: El caso Ezpeleta*. Buenos Aires: La Marca Editora.

Chatterjee, Partha. 2006. *The Politics of the Governed*. New York: Columbia University Press.

Ciudad Autónoma de Buenos Aires. 2008. *Guía de servicios sociales: Ministerio de Desarrollo Social*. Buenos Aires: Gobierno de la Ciudad de Buenos Aires.

Cohen, Stanley, and Laurie Taylor. 1972. *Psychological Survival: The Experience of Long-Term Imprisonment*. Middlesex, U.K.: Penguin.

Colomy, Paul, and David Brown. 1996. "Goffman and Interactional Citizenship." *Sociological Perspectives* 39 (3): 371–81.

Comfort, Megan. 2008. *Doing Time Together*. Chicago: University of Chicago Press.

Comisión Provincial por la Memoria. 2010. *Violaciones a los derechos humanos en los lugares de detención de la provincia de Buenos Aires*. Buenos Aires: Comisión Provincial por la Memoria.

Cooney, Paul. 2007. "Argentina's Quarter-Century Experiment with Neo-liberalism: From Dictatorship to Depression." *Revista de Economia Contemporânea* 11 (1): 7–37.

Corte Suprema de Justicia (CSJ). 2008. "Mendoza Beatriz Silvia and Others v. the National State and Others Regarding Damages Suffered (Injuries Resulting from the Environmental Contamination of the Matanza-Riachuelo River)." Fundación Ambiente y Recursos Naturales, http://www.farn.org.ar/.

Cravino, María Cristina. 2006. *Las villas de la ciudad: Mercado e informalidad urbana*. Los Polvorines, Argentina: Universidad de General Sarmiento.

Cravino, María Cristina, Juan Pablo del Rio, and Juan Ignacio Duarte. 2008. "Magnitud y crecimiento de las villas y asentamientos en el área aetropolitana de Buenos Aires en los últimos 25 años." Paper presented at the XIV Encuentro de la Red Universitaria Latinoamericana de Cátedras de Vivienda—Facultad de Arquitectura, Urbanismo y Diseño—Universidad de Buenos Aires. October 1–4, 2008. www.fadu.uba.ar/.

Daroqui, Alcira, Carlos Motos, Ana Laura Lopez. 2009. *Muertes silenciadas*. Buenos Aires: Centro Cultural de la Cooperación.

Das, Veena, ed. 1990. *Mirrors of Violence: Communities, Riots, and Survivors in South Asia*. Oxford: Oxford University Press.

Davis, Mike. 2006. *Planet of Slums*. London: Verso.

Defensoría de la Ciudad de Buenos Aires. n.d. "Los desalojos y la emergencia habitacional en la ciudad de Buenos Aires." http://www.defensoria.org.ar/.

——. 2009. *El Derecho a la vivienda.* http://www.defensoria.org.ar/.

Defensoría del Pueblo de la Nación Argentina. 2003. *Informe especial sobre la cuenca Matanza-Riachuelo.* Buenos Aires: Defensoría del Pueblo de la Nación Argentina.

——. 2009. "Los efectos de la contaminación ambiental en la niñez. Una cuestión de derechos." http://www.defensor.gov.ar/.

Dorado, Carlos. 2006. "Informe sobre Dock Sud." Unpublished manuscript.

Durkheim, Emile. 1965. *The Elementary Forms of Religious Life.* New York: Free Press.

Eckstein, Susan, ed. 2001. *Power and Popular Protest: Latin American Social Movements.* Berkeley: University of California Press.

Edelman, Marc. 2001. "Social Movements: Changing Paradigms and Forms of Politics." *Annual Review of Anthropology* 30: 285–317.

Edin, Katherine, and Laura Lein. 1997. *Making Ends Meet: How Single Mothers Survive Welfare and Low-Wage Work.* New York: Russell Sage Foundation.

Ehrenreich, Barbara. 2001. *Nickel and Dimed: On (Not) Getting By in America.* New York: Holt.

Emirbayer, Mustafa, and Ann Mische. 1998. "What Is Agency?" *American Journal of Sociology* 103: 962–1023.

Engels, Friedrich. 1973 [1844]. *The Condition of the Working-Class in England.* London: Lawrence and Wishart.

Epele, María. 2010. *Sujetar por la herida: Una etnografía sobre drogas, pobreza y salud.* Buenos Aires: Paidós.

Flaherty, Michael. 1999. *A Watched Pot: How We Experience Time.* New York: New York University Press.

——. 2010. *The Textures of Time: Agency and Temporal Experience.* Philadelphia: Temple University Press.

Flaherty, Michael, Betina Freidin, and Ruth Sautu. 2005. "Variation in the Perceived Passage of Time: A Cross-National Study." *Social Psychology Quarterly* 68: 400–410.

Foucault, Michel. 1979. *Discipline and Punish.* New York: Vintage.

——. 1991. "Governmentality." *The Foucault Effect: Studies in Governmentality,* edited by Graham Burchell, Colin Gordon, and Peter Miller, 87–104. Chicago: University of Chicago Press.

——. 2000. *Power: Essential Works of Foucault, 1954–1984.* New York: New Press.

Fraser, Nancy. 1989. *Unruly Practices.* Minneapolis: University of Minnesota Press.

——. 1990. "Struggle over Needs: Outline of a Socialist-Feminist Critical Theory of Late-Capitalist Political Culture." *Women, the State, and Welfare,* edited by Linda Gordon, 199–225. Madison: University of Wisconsin Press.

Fundación Ambiente y Recursos Naturales (FARN). 2009. *Annual Environmental Report*. Buenos Aires: Fundación Ambiente y Recursos Naturales. http://www.farn.org.ar/.

García Márquez, Gabriel. 1979 [1961]. *No One Writes to the Colonel*. New York: Harper and Row.

Garfinkel, Harold. 1967. *Studies in Ethnomethodology*. Englewood Cliffs, N.J.: Prentice-Hall.

Garland, David, ed. 2006. *Mass Imprisonment: Social Causes and Consequences*. London: Sage.

Gasparini, Giovanni. 1995. "On Waiting." *Time and Society* 4 (1): 29–45.

Gaventa, John. 1980. *Power and Powerlessness: Quiescence and Rebellion in an Appalachian Valley*. Champaign: University of Illinois Press.

Gay, Robert. 1994. *Popular Organization and Democracy in Rio de Janeiro: A Tale of Two Favelas*. Philadelphia: Temple University Press.

Geertz, Clifford. 1973. *The Interpretation of Cultures*. New York: Basic Books.

Giarracca, Norma, ed. 2001. *La protesta social en la Argentina: Transformaciones económicas y crisis social en el interior del país*. Buenos Aires: Alianza Editorial.

Giddens, Anthony. 1986. *The Constitution of Society*. New York: Polity Press.

Gilliom, John. 2001. *Overseers of the Poor*. Chicago: University of Chicago Press.

Gilman, Richard. 1987. "The Waiting Since." *Samuel Beckett's Waiting for Godot*, edited by Harold Bloom, 67–78. New York: Chelsea House.

Giraudy, Agustina. 2007. "The Distributive Politics of Emergency Employment Programs in Argentina." *Latin American Research Review* 42 (2): 33–55.

Goffman, Alice. 2009. "On the Run: Wanted Men in a Philadelphia Ghetto." *American Sociological Review* 74 (3): 339–57.

Goffman, Erving. 1952. "On Cooling the Mark Out: Some Aspects of Adaptation to Failure." *Psychiatry* 15 (4): 451–63.

———. 1961. *Encounters: Two Studies in the Sociology of Interaction*. New York: Macmillan.

Goldberg, Chad. 2007. *Citizens and Paupers*. Chicago: University of Chicago Press.

Goldstein, Donna. 1998. "Nothing Bad Intended: Child Discipline, Punishment, and Survival in a Shantytown in Rio de Janeiro, Brazil." *Small Wars: The Cultural Politics of Childhood*, edited by Nancy Scheper-Hughes and Carolyn Sargent, 389–415. Berkeley: University of California Press.

———. 2003. *Laughter Out of Place: Race, Class, and Sexuality in a Rio Shantytown*. Berkeley: University of California Press.

Goodsell, Charles. 1984. "Welfare Waiting Rooms." *Urban Life* 12: 467–77.

Gorban, Débora. 2006. "Experiencia y representaciones de una actividad particular: El caso de las mujeres cartoneras del Tren Blanco." Paper presented

at VIII Jornadas Nacionales de Historia de las Mujeres III Congreso
Iberoamericano de Estudios de Genero. Villa Giardino, Córdoba.

———. 2009. "Restituyendo tramas: Cuando la carreta es más que la 'última
opción.'" Paper presented at VIII Reunión de Antropología del MER-
COSUR, "Diversidad y Poder en América Latina," UNSAM, Buenos Aires,
Argentina.

Gordon, Linda, ed. 1990a. *Women, the State, and Welfare*. Madison: University
of Wisconsin Press.

———. 1990b. "The New Feminist Scholarship on the Welfare State." *Women,
the State, and Welfare*, edited by Linda Gordon, 9–35. Madison: University of
Wisconsin Press.

Guerra, Nancy, Rowell Huesmann, and Anja Spindler. 2003. "Community Violence Exposure, Social Cognition and Aggression among Urban Elementary
School Children." *Child Development* 74 (5): 1561–76.

Gupta, Akhil. 1995. "Blurred Boundaries: The Discourse of Corruption, the
Culture of Politics, and the Imagined State." *American Ethnologist* 22 (2):
375–402.

———. 2005. "Narratives of Corruption: Anthropological and Fictional
Accounts of the Indian State." *Ethnography* 6 (1): 5–34.

Hall, Edward T. 1959. *The Silent Language*. New York: Anchor Books.

Haney, Lynne. 1996. "Homeboys, Babies, and Men in Suits: The State and the
Reproduction of Male Dominance." *American Sociological Review* 61 (5):
759–78.

Harvey, David. 2005. *A Brief History of Neoliberalism*. New York: Oxford University Press.

Hasenfeld, Y. 1972. "People Processing Organizations: An Exchange
Approach." *American Sociological Review* 37: 256–63.

Hays, Sharon. 2003. *Flat Broke with Children. Women in the Age of Welfare
Reform*. New York: Oxford University Press.

Heller, Patrick, and Peter Evans. 2010. "Taking Tilly South: Durable Inequalities, Democratic Contestation, and Citizenship in the Southern Metropolis."
Theory and Society 39: 433–50.

Hochschild, Arlie Russell. 2001. *The Time Bind*. New York: Holt.

Holston, James. 2008. *Insurgent Citizenship*. Princeton: Princeton University
Press.

Holzner, Claudio. 2004. "The End of Clientelism? Strong and Weak Networks
in a Mexican Squatter Movement." *Mobilization* 9 (3): 223–40.

Hoshaw, Lindsey. 2008. "Troubled Waters: The Matanza-Riachuelo River
Basin." The Argentina Independent. http://www.argentinaindependent
.com/.

Instituto Nacional de Estadísticas y Censos (INDEC). 2003. "Incidencia de la pobreza y de la indigencia en el Gran Buenos Aires, Mayo 2003." http://www.indec.gov.ar/.

Jacobs, Jerry, and Kathleen Gerson. 2005. *The Time Divide*. Cambridge: Harvard University Press.

Jessop, Bob. 1999. "Narrating the Future of the National Economy and the National State: Remarks on Remapping Regulation and Reinventing Governance." *State/Culture: State Formation after the Cultural Turn*, edited by George Steinmetz, 378–406. Ithaca: Cornell University Press.

Jin, Ha. 2000. *Waiting: A Novel*. New York: Vintage.

JMB Ingeniería Ambiental. 2003. "Plan de Acción Estratégico para la Gestión Ambiental Sustentable de un Area Urbano-Industrial a Escala Completa" (PAE). Informe Final.

Johnston, Hank, and Paul D. Almeida, eds. 2006. *Latin American Social Movements: Globalization, Democratization, and Transnational Networks*. Lanham, Md.: Rowman and Littlefield.

Joseph, Gilbert, and Daniel Nugent, eds. 1994. *Everyday Forms of State Formation*. Durham: Duke University Press.

Kafka, Franz. 1998 [1946]. *The Trial*. New York: Schocken Books.

Katz, Jack. 1982. *Poor People's Lawyers in Transition*. New Brunswick: Rutgers University Press.

Kenner, Hugh. 1987. "Waiting for Godot." *Samuel Beckett's Waiting for Godot*, edited by Harold Bloom, 53–66. New York: Chelsea House Publishers.

Kerkvliet, Ben T. 2005. *The Power of Everyday Politics: How Vietnamese Peasants Transformed National Policy*. Ithaca: Cornell University Press.

Kirschke, Linda. 2000. "Informal Repression: Zero-Sum Politics and Late Third Wave Transitions." *Journal of Modern African Studies* 38 (3): 383–403.

Kohen, Beatriz, Carmen Hernáez, Diego Kravetz, Andrés Nápoli, and Mabel Romero. 2001. "El control ciudadano del derecho a un medio ambiente sano en la Ciudad de Buenos Aires y su área metropolitana: Aspectos ambientales y jurídico-institucionales." Fundación Ambiente y Recursos Naturales, Buenos Aires.

Koonings, Kees. 2001. "Armed Actors, Violence and Democracy in Latin America in the 1990s." *Bulletin of Latin American Research* 20 (4): 401–8.

Korbin, Jill. 2003. "Children, Childhoods, and Violence." *Annual Review of Anthropology* 32: 431–46.

Korteweg, Anna. 2006. "The Construction of Gendered Citizenship at the Welfare Office: An Ethnographic Comparison of Welfare-to-Work Workshops in the United States and the Netherlands." *Social Politics* 13 (3): 313–40.

Lamont, Michelle, and Virag Molnár. 2002. "The Study of Boundaries across the Social Sciences." *Annual Review of Sociology* 28: 167–95.

Lazar, Sian. 2008. *El Alto, Rebel City: Self and Citizenship in Andean Bolivia.* Durham: Duke University Press.

Lens, Vicki. 2007. "Administrative Justice in Public Welfare Bureaucracies. When Citizens (Don't) Complain." *Administration and Society* 39 (3): 382–408.

Levine, Robert. 1997. *A Geography of Time.* New York: Basic Books.

Lichterman, Paul. 1998. "What Do Movements Mean? The Value of Participant Observation." *Qualitative Sociology* 21: 401–18.

Lipsky, Michael. 1980. *Street-Level Bureaucracy.* New York: Russell Sage Foundation.

——. 1984. "Bureaucratic Disentitlement in Social Welfare Programs." *Social Service Review* 58 (1): 3–27.

Lipsky, Michael, and Steven Rathgeb Smith. 1989. "When Social Problems are Treated as Emergencies." *Social Service Review* 63 (1): 5–25.

Lukes, Steven. 2004. *Power: A Radical View.* New York: Palgrave.

MacLeod, Jay. 1995. *Ain't No Making It: Aspirations and Attainment in a Low-Income Neighborhood.* Boulder, Colo.: Westview Press.

Mann, Leon. 1969. "Queue Culture: The Waiting Line as a Social System." *American Journal of Sociology* 75: 340–54.

Margolin, Gayla, and Elana Gordis. 2000. "The Effects of Family and Community Violence on Children." *Annual Review of Psychology* 51: 445–79.

Markowitz, Gerald, and David Rosner. 2002. *Deceit and Denial. The Deadly Politics of Industrial Pollution.* Berkeley: University of California Press.

Marx, Karl. 1887. *Capital.* Vol. 1. New York: New World.

Mauer, Marc, and Meda Chesney-Lind. 2002. *Invisible Punishment: The Collateral Consequences of Mass Imprisonment.* New York: New Press.

McCart, Michael, Daniel Smith, Benjamin Saunders, Dean Kilpatrick, Heidi Resnick, and Kenneth Ruggiero. 2007. "Do Urban Adolescents Become Desensitized to Community Violence? Data from National Survey." *American Journal of Orthopsychiatry* 77 (3): 434–42.

Merton, Robert K. 1987. "Three Fragments from a Sociologist's Notebooks: Establishing the Phenomenon, Specified Ignorance, and Strategic Research Materials." *Annual Review of Sociology* 13: 1–28.

Mink, Gwendolyn. 1990. "The Lady and the Tramp: Gender, Race, and the Origins of the American Welfare State." *Women, the State, and Welfare,* edited by Linda Gordon, 99–122. Madison: University of Wisconsin Press.

Mirowsky, John, and Catherine E. Ross. 1983. "Paranoia and the Structure of Powerlessness." *American Sociological Review* 48 (2): 228–39.

Mulcahy, Caitlin, Diana C. Parry, and Troy D. Glover. 2010. "The 'Patient Patient': The Trauma of Waiting and the Power of Resistance for People Living with Cancer." *Qualitative Health Research* 20 (8): 1062–75.

Müller, Markus-Michael. 2012. "The Rise of the Penal State in Latin America." *Contemporary Justice Review*. Forthcoming.

Munn, Nancy. 1992. "The Cultural Anthropology of Time: A Critical Essay." *Annual Review of Anthropology* 21: 91–123.

Navarro, Marysa, and Nicholas Fraser. 1985. *Eva Perón*. New York: Norton.

Nelson, Barbara. 1990. "The Origins of the Two-Channel Welfare State: Workmen's Compensations and Mothers' Aid." *Women, the State, and Welfare*, edited by Linda Gordon, 123–51. Madison: University of Wisconsin Press.

Nun, José. 2001. *Marginalidad y Exclusión Social*. Buenos Aires: Fondo de Cultura Económica.

O'Brien, Edna. 1995. "Waiting." *The Best American Essays*, edited by J. Kincaid and R. Atawan, 38–46. Boston: Houghton Mifflin Company.

O'Donnell, Guilermo. 1993. "On the State, Democratization and Some Conceptual Problems: A Latin American View with Glances at Some Postcommunist Countries." *World Development* 21: 1355–69.

Orloff, Ann Shola. 1999. "Motherhood, Work, and Welfare in the United States, Britain, Canada, and Australia." *State/Culture: State Formation after the Cultural Turn*, edited by George Steinmetz, 321–54. Ithaca: Cornell University Press.

Ortner, Sherry. 2006. *Anthropology and Social Theory*. Durham: Duke University Press.

Oszlak, Oscar. 1991. *Merecer la ciudad: Los pobres y el derecho al espacio urbano*. Buenos Aires: Humanitas.

Partnoy, Alicia. 1998. *The Little School: Tales of Disappearance and Survival in Argentina*. San Francisco: Cleiss Press.

Pateman, Carole. 1988. "The Patriarchal Welfare State." *Democracy and the Welfare State*, edited by A. Gutmann, 231–60. Princeton: Princeton University Press.

Pearce, Jenny. 2010. "Perverse State Formation and Securitized Democracy in Latin America." *Democratization* 17 (2): 286–306.

Peck, Jamie, and Adam Tickell. 2002. "Neoliberalizing Space." *Antipode* 34 (3): 380–404.

Perlman, Janice. 1976. *The Myth of Marginality*. Berkeley: University of California Press.

———. 2010. *Favela: Four Decades of Living on the Edge in Rio de Janeiro*. New York: Oxford University Press.

Pírez, Pedro. 2001. "Buenos Aires: Fragmentation and Privatization of the Metropolitan City." *Environment and Urbanization* 14 (1): 145–58.

Piven, Frances, and Richard Cloward. 1971. *Regulating the Poor: The Functions of Public Welfare*. New York: Vintage.

———. 1978. *Poor People's Movements*. New York: Vintage.

Portes Alejandro, and Bryan R. Roberts. 2005. "The Free-Market City: Latin American Urbanization in the Years of the Neoliberal Experiment." *Studies in Comparative International Development* 40 (1): 43–82.

Procupez, Valeria, and Maria Carla Rodriguez. 2001. "Bringing It All Back Home: Homelessness and Alternative Housing Policies among Urban Squatters in Buenos Aires, Argentina." *International Perspectives on Homelessness*, edited by Valerie Polakow and Cindy Guillean, 216–40. Westport, Conn.: Greenwood Press.

Prottas, Jeffrey. 1979. *People Processing: The Street-Level Bureaucrat in Public Service Bureaucracies*. New York: Lexington Books.

Purser, Gretchen. 2006. "Waiting for Work: An Ethnography of a Day Labor Agency." University of California, Berkeley, Institute for the Study of Social Change. http://www.escholarship.org/.

Rabinow, Paul, ed. 1984. *Foucault: A Reader*. New York: Pantheon.

Redko, Cristina, Richard Rapp, and Robert Carlson. 2006. "Waiting Time as a Barrier to Treatment Entry: Perceptions of Substance Abusers." *Journal of Drug Issues* 22: 831–52.

Revista Mu. 2008. "Barrios Cerrados: La Militarización de La Cava." (March): 10–11.

Robinson, William. 2008. *Latin America and Global Capitalism: A Critical Globalization Perspective*. Baltimore: Johns Hopkins University Press.

Roseberry, William. 1994. "Hegemony and the Language of Contention." *Everyday Forms of State Formation*, edited by Gilbert Joseph and Daniel Nugent, 355–66. Durham: Duke University Press.

Roth, Julius. 1963. *Timetables: Structuring the Passage of Time in Hospital Treatment and Other Careers*. Indianapolis: Bobbs-Merrill.

Rotstein, Dalia, and David Alter. 2006. "Where Does the Waiting List Begin? A Short Review of the Dynamics and Organization of Modern Waiting Lists." *Social Science and Medicine* 62: 3157–60.

Roy, Beth. 1994. *Some Trouble with Cows: Making Sense of Social Conflict*. Berkeley: University of California Press.

Roy, Donald. 1959. "Banana Time: Job Satisfaction and Informal Interaction." *Human Organization* 18: 158–68.

Salvia, Agustín. 2007. "Consideraciones sobre la transición a la modernidad, la exclusión social y la marginalidad económica: Un campo abierto a la investigación social y al debate político." *Sombras de una marginalidad fragmentada: Aproximaciones a la metamorfosis de los sectores populares de la Argentina*, edited by Agustín Salvia and Eduardo Chávez Molina, 25–66. Buenos Aires: Miño y Dávila.

Salvia, Agustín, and Eduardo Chávez Molina, eds. 2007. *Sombras de una marginalidad fragmentada. Aproximaciones a la metamorfosis de los sectores populares de la Argentina*. Buenos Aires: Miño y Dávila.

Sayer, Derek. 1994. "Everyday Forms of State Formation: Some Dissident Remarks on 'Hegemony.' " *Everyday Forms of State Formation*, edited by Gilbert Joseph and Daniel Nugent, 367–77. Durham: Duke University Press.

Schatz, Edward, ed. 2009. *Political Ethnography: What Immersion Contributes to the Study of Power*. Chicago: University of Chicago Press.

Scheper-Hughes, Nancy. 1992. *Death without Weeping*. Berkeley: University of California Press.

Scheper-Hughes, Nancy, and Philippe Bourgois, eds. 2004. *Violence in War and Peace*. Malden, Mass.: Blackwell.

Schutz, Alfred. 1964. *The Problem of Social Reality: Collected Papers 1*. The Hague: Martinus Nijhoff.

Schwartz, Barry. 1974. "Waiting, Exchange, and Power: The Distribution of Time in Social Systems." *American Journal of Sociology* 79: 841–70.

——. 1975. *Queuing and Waiting: Studies in the Social Organization of Access and Delay*. Chicago: University of Chicago Press.

Schweizer, Howard. 2008. *On Waiting*. London: Routledge.

Scott, James. 1990. *Domination and the Art of Resistance: Hidden Transcripts*. New Haven: Yale University Press.

——. 1999. *Seeing like the State*. New Haven: Yale University Press.

Scott, James, and Ben Kerkvliet. 1977. "How Traditional Rural Patrons Lose Legitimacy: A Theory with Special Reference to Southeast Asia." *Friends, Followers, and Factions: A Reader in Political Clientelism*, edited by Steffen W. Schmidt, James C. Scott, Carl Lande, and Laura Guasti, 439–58. Berkeley: University of California Press.

Secor, Anna. 2007. "Between Longing and Despair: State, Space and Subjectivity in Turkey." *Environment and Planning D: Society and Space* 25: 33–52.

Shaheed, Farida. 1990. "The Pathan-Muhajir Conflicts, 1985–6: A National Perspective." *Mirrors of Violence: Communities, Riots and Survivors in South Asia*, edited by Veena Das, 194–214. Oxford: Oxford University Press.

Shefner, Jon. 2008. *The Illusion of Civil Society: Democratization and Community Mobilization in Low-Income Mexico*. University Park: Pennsylvania State University Press.

Small, Mario Luis, David J. Harding, and Michele Lamont. 2010. "Reconsidering Culture and Poverty." *Annals of the American Academy of Political and Social Science* 629: 6–27.

Sorokin, Pitirim, and Robert Merton. 1937. "Social Time: A Methodological and Functional Analysis." *American Journal of Sociology* 42: 615–29.

Sorokin, Vladimir. 2008. *The Queue*. New York: New York Review of Books.

Soss, Joe. 1999. "Welfare Application Encounters: Subordination, Satisfaction, and the Puzzle of Client Evaluations." *Administration and Society* 31 (1): 50–94.

Steinmetz, George, ed. 1999. Introduction to *State/Culture: State Formation after the Cultural Turn*. 1–50. Ithaca: Cornell University Press.

Svampa, Maristella. 2001. *Los que ganaron: La vida en los countries y barrios privados*. Buenos Aires: Editorial Biblos.

Svampa, Maristella, and Sebastián Pereyra. 2003. *Entre la ruta y el barrio: La experiencia de las organizaciones piqueteras*. Buenos Aires: Editorial Biblos.

Tarrow, Sidney. 1996. "The People's Two Rhythms: Charles Tilly and the Study of Contentious Politics." *Comparative Studies in Society and History* 38: 586–600.

Teubal, Miguel. 2004. "Rise and Collapse of Neoliberalism in Argentina: The Role of Economic Groups." *Journal of Developing Societies* 20 (3–4): 173–88.

Thompson, Edward P. 1994. *Customs in Common*. New York: New Press.

Thompson, Jeffery, and Stuart Bunderson. 2001. "Work-Nonwork Conflict and the Phenomenology of Time: Beyond the Balance Metaphor." *Work and Occupations* 28 (1): 17–39.

Tilly, Charles. 1985. "War Making and State Making as Organized Crime." *Bringing the State Back In*, edited by Peter Evans, Dietrich Rueschemeyer, and Theda Skocpol, 169–91. New York: Cambridge University Press.

———. ed. 1997a. *Roads from Past to Future*. Lanham, Md.: Rowman and Littlefield.

———. 1997b. "Invisible Elbows." *Roads from Past to Future*, edited by Charles Tilly, 35–48. Lanham, Md.: Rowman and Littlefield.

———. 2003. *The Politics of Collective Violence*. New York: Cambridge University Press.

———. 2006. *Regimes and Repertoires*. Chicago: Chicago University Press.

———. 2007. *Democracy*. New York: Cambridge University Press.

———. 2008. *Credit and Blame*. Princeton: Princeton University Press.

Ungar, Mark, and Ana Laura Magaloni. 2009. "Latin America's Prisons: A Crisis of Criminal Policy and Democratic Rule." *Criminality, Public Security, and the Challenge to Democracy in Latin America*, edited by Marcelo Bergman and Laurence Whitehead, 223–48. Notre Dame, Ind.: University of Notre Dame Press.

United Nations Environment Programme (UNEP); United Nations Children's Fund (UNICEF). 1997. *Childhood Poisoning: Information for Advocacy and Action*. New York: UNEP-UNICEF.

United Nations Human Settlements Programme. 2003. *The Challenge of Slums: Global Report on Human Settlements 2003*. London: Earthscan Publications.

Varshney, Ashutosh. 2002. *Ethnic Conflict and Civic Life: Hindus and Muslims in India*. New Haven: Yale University Press.

Vaughan, Diane. 2004. "Theorizing Disaster: Analogy, Historical Ethnography, and the Challenger Accident." *Ethnography* 5 (3): 315–47.

Venkatesh, Sudhir. 2002. "'Doin' the Hustle': Constructing the Ethnographer in the American Ghetto." *Ethnography* 3 (1): 91–111.

Verbitsky, Horacio. 2010. "Los treinta mil." June 27. Página12, www.pagina12.com.ar/.

Villalón, Roberta. 2007. "Neoliberalism, Corruption, and Legacies of Contention: Argentina's Social Movements, 1993–2006." *Latin American Perspectives* 34 (2): 139–56.

Wacquant, Loïc. 1995. "The Comparative Structure and Experience of Urban Exclusion: 'Race,' Class, and Space in Chicago and Paris." *Poverty, Inequality and the Future of Social Policy*, edited by Katherine McFate, Roger Lawson, and William Julius Wilson, 543–70. New York: Russell Sage Foundation.

———. 1998. "Negative Social Capital: State Breakdown and Social Destitution in America's Urban Core." *Netherlands Journal of Housing and the Built Environment* 13: 25–39.

———. 2002. "Scrutinizing the Street: Poverty, Morality, and the Pitfalls of Urban Ethnography." *American Journal of Sociology* 107 (6): 1468–532.

———. 2003a. *Body and Soul*. New York: Oxford University Press.

———. 2003b. "Ethnografeast: A Progress Report on the Practice and Promise of Ethnography." *Ethnography* 4: 5–14.

———. 2008. "Ordering Insecurity: Social Polarization and the Punitive Upsurge." *Radical Philosophy Review* 11 (1): 9–27.

———. 2009. *Punishing the Poor: The Neoliberal Government of Social Insecurity*. Durham: Duke University Press.

Watkins-Hays, Celeste. 2009. *The New Welfare Bureaucrats*. Chicago: University of Chicago Press.

Weber, Max. 1978. *Economy and Society*. Berkeley: University of California Press.

Wedeen, Lisa. 1999. *Ambiguities of Domination*. Chicago: University of Chicago Press.

Weitz-Shapiro, Rebecca. 2008. "Choosing Clientelism." Ph.D. dissertation, Columbia University.

Western, Bruce. 2006. *Punishment and Inequality in America*. New York: Russell Sage Foundation.

Wilding, Polly. 2010. "'New Violence': Silencing Women's Experiences in the Favelas of Brazil." *Journal of Latin American Studies* 42: 719–47.

Wilkinson, Steven. 2004. *Votes and Violence: Electoral Competition and Ethnic Riots in India*. Cambridge: Cambridge University Press.

Willis, Paul. 1977. *Learning to Labor*. New York: Columbia University Press.

Wolford, Wendy. 2010. *The Land Is Ours Now*. Durham: Duke University Press.

Wood, Elisabeth Jean. 2003. *Insurgent Collective Action and Civil War in El Salvador*. New York: Cambridge University Press.

Yang, Shu-Yuan. 2005. "Imagining the State: An Ethnographic Study." *Ethnography* 6 (4): 487–516.

Young, Alford. 2004. *The Minds of Marginalized Black Men*. Princeton: Princeton University Press.

Zerubavel, Eviatar. 1979. *Patterns of Time in Hospital Life*. Chicago: University of Chicago Press.

Zolberg, Aristide. 1972. "Moments of Madness." *Politics and Society* 2: 183–207.

INDEX

JAVIER AUYERO is Joe R. and Teresa Lozano Long Professor of Latin American Sociology at the University of Texas, Austin.

Library of Congress Cataloging-in-Publication Data
Auyero, Javier.
Patients of the state : the politics of waiting in Argentina / Javier Auyero.
p. cm.
Includes bibliographical references and index.
ISBN 978-0-8223-5259-4 (cloth : alk. paper)
ISBN 978-0-8223-5233-4 (pbk. : alk. paper)
1. Poor—Services for—Argentina. 2. Poor—Government policy—Argentina.
3. Poverty—Argentina. 4. Marginality, Social—Argentina. I. Title.
HC180.P6A99 2012
362.5'560982—dc23
2011035892